MW01595591

Archbishop Lazar Puhalo

THE IMPACT OF BYZANTINE CHRISTIAN THOUGHT ON MEDICINE.

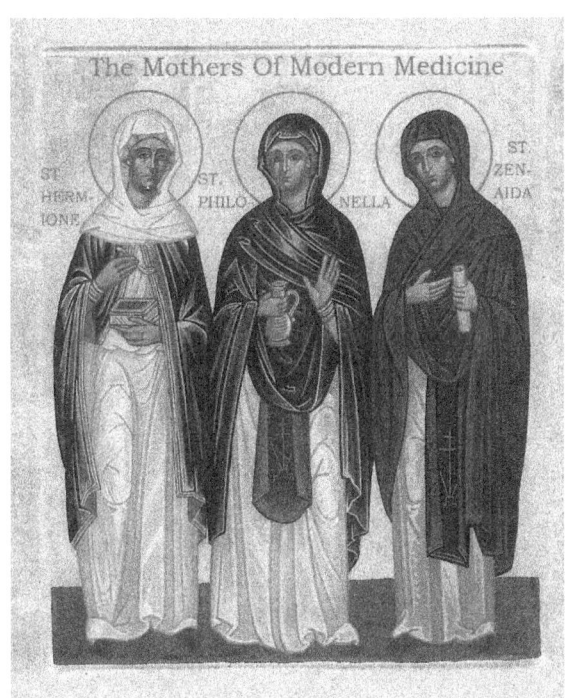

The Mothers Of Modern Medicine

ST. HERMIONE · ST. PHILONELLA · ST. ZENAIDA

SYNAXIS PRESS
P.O. BOX 18
DEWDNEY, BC
CANADA, V0M-1H0

ISBN: 978-1974179046
COPYRIGHT 1974
Synaxis Press
(This book is an expansion of a paper presented at an
international conference on Religion and Medicine spon-
sored by the University of Alberta)

CONTENTS

1
SYNOPSIS

In the first several centuries of the Christian era, medicine developed more rapidly in the East than in the Latin West. The author of this book presents the suggestion that, in great part, the difference lies in the respective concepts of what actually constitutes the human person. The radical difference between East and West, in the understanding of redemption also played an important role in this phenomenon. There was also a difference in the understanding of the Epistles of Apostle Paul. From the time of Augustine of Hippo, neo-platonism began to dominate Latin theological systems. More attention was given to the punishment of man than to his healing. In the words of the Roman Catholic theologian Karl Rahner:

> *The East thought in terms of a dynamic*
> *saving history and an ascending order of*
> *things, beginning with the economy of*
> *the Trinity and closely bound up with*

soteriology. Redemption is regarded in the East as a real ontological process that begins with the incarnation, discloses the immanent economy of the Trinity, ends with the divinization [theosis] of the world and first proves its triumph in Christ's Resurrection. In contrast, Western theology regards the incarnation of The Logos almost exclusively as the means of constituting a fit agent capable of making satisfaction for sin. Though aware of the divinization [theosis] of the world, it lays much more stress on Christ's atonement for sin on the Cross and on forgiveness.[1]

While the Orthodox Christian Church was convinced of the unity of body and soul, which mutually complement each other, the Latin West became influenced by the Gnostic and Platonistic concept of "dualism"— the idea of a radical dichotomy between body and soul in the human person.

This Gnostic idea tends to see an enmity between body and soul, indeed, between the material and that which is said to be spiritual. It conveys the idea that the body is a prison of the soul, and that the soul is *liberated* from the body by death (or, at least partly, by extreme asceticism), whereupon, it experiences new freedom, rises to new heights, experiences new discoveries and wanders freely now that it is, according to Gnosticism, free of its sinful body. This concept likely arose from a lack of knowledge about the function of the brain and mind. Since the body responds to the activity of the brain – to thoughts and desires of the mind – it was felt that the body acted autonomously in a manner that was contrary to the higher spiritual efforts of the *nous* (mind/soul/intellect). In Gnostic thought, the body and soul are seen as completely separate entities and, indeed, in many of the Gnostic sects, the soul was thought to have a "subtle physical body"[2] of its own. This is the source of the unscriptural notion that the soul of a deceased person becomes an angel (as one often sees in Western cartoons or other illustrations), with a complete, though subtle, physical body in which it can experience new things, endure trials at the hands of archon/demons, and inherit paradise or gehenna alone, without the body, before the general resurrection. Such an idea negates the general resurrection, as well as the Second Coming and Last Judgment by Christ.

In some extreme cases, the Gnostic and Augustinian neo-Platonists concluded that, since the soul has a "subtle body," the general resurrection is only metaphorical, for there would be no reason for God to reunite the soul with its old enemy, the body.

Among the Gnostic sects and neo-Platonists, there developed a separate "ascetic theology" which is generally at odds with major principles of the "patristic theology" of the great Church fathers. The very term "ascetic theology" can often be a synonym for "Gnostic sect."

The development of bio-medicine (and of the

psychological sciences) was greatly hindered by such concepts, because the body was conceived as being at odds with the soul, and therefore had to be treated separately, and in a lesser manner or not at all. Thus, while hospitals developed as medical centres in the East, in the West they remained largely palliative care hospices until quite late. Active research into physical illnesses and their treatments was not so important, since the destruction of the body was beneficial for the soul. Some element of this idea of dualism was still present when Descartes (1596-1650) erroneously separated the mind from the body and asserted that the body could function quite well without the mind.[3] Such dualism appears also in the epistemology of John Locke, one of the fathers of modern democracy, as well in the thought of several other Western philosophers. From them, it entered into the general consciousness of the West. Protestantism appears not to have comprehended the danger of such teachings.

In the Orthodox Christian concept, expressed by the holy fathers, soul and body are a single, harmonious unit which together make up the "person" – the human being. Thus, treatment of the illnesses of both soul and body were equally sacred acts and desirable. Christ Himself often cured one by treating the other. Thus, the healing of a bodily infirmity might be accomplished by the forgiveness of sins *(Mt. 9:2-7)*. Christ and, following Him, the saints of the Orthodox Church had the concept of what in our own time is called "holistic medicine."

It is interesting that even the concept of a so-called "*partial* judgment"[4] at death and the "actual judgment" upon resurrection, directly reflects this Orthodox concept, so important to scientific medicine, of the unity of soul and body. The *person* cannot be judged and rewarded when he is dissolved into two components, body separate from soul. Therefore, the soul, which remains alive at the death of the body is only a *part* of the person, but not the person, and so it can only be assigned to a state proper to itself at death, that is, a condition of joyous expectation or of dread. No judgment can be passed or rewards received until, in the resurrection, soul and body are reunited as the "person." This "assignment" of the soul is called a "partial" judgment precisely because it is dealing with only a *part* of the person. The Orthodox Church fathers are especially adamant in declaring that the soul alone is not the person, nor is the body.[5] Thus, there is a "partial" judgment, which consists only in the soul becoming aware of its condition and the destiny it will share with the body in the resurrection, and an *actual* judgment can come about only when the reunion of soul and body restores the actual person.

Gnostic sects are inclined to the pagan idea that the soul, having, as they suppose, a "subtle physical body" of its own, actually constitutes the complete person, and the body is only fictionally necessary. While this Gnosticism appears periodically among some monastic writers in the Orthodox Church (usually those under the influence of Augustinianism), it actually entered into the general theology of the Latin West. There one can also trace it to the influence of Plato's *Timaeus* and *Phaedros*.

According to Amanda Porterfield, "Commitment to a holistic Christian society was strong in the East. Beginning in the fourth century, Eastern bishops urged citizens to construct a virtuous society, dedicated to the common good and to the welfare of the sick and poor."[6] Historian Timothy Miller says that "Eastern bishops came to see the practice of *philanthropia*,[7] as a force which aimed at transforming the pagan world, represented by the ancient *polis*, into a truly Christian society, a heavenly city."[8]

"In recasting the ancient Greek ideal of a strong, unified, and virtuous polis in Christian terms," adds John Meyendorff:

> *Eastern churchmen supported the interdependence of church and Empire and the emperor's obligation to act as God's emissary, at the same time emphasizing*

man's free will and potential for deification. In some contrast, Augustine and other churchmen affiliated with Rome emphasized the innate sinfulness of human beings and the need for obedience to rulers authorized by God to control and punish human behaviour. For reasons both theological and practical, churchmen in the West were less idealistic about Christian society, more pessimistic about human nature.[9]

As a result of more holistic and optimistic thinking about Christian society in Eastern Christianity, medicine developed as an aspect and necessary manifestation of the Orthodox faith.

Eventually, the medical theories of the ancient Hellenic physician Galen were dogmatized, rather than built upon, in the West. As a result of the eventual exposure to the medical and scientific theories of the Islamic schools in Moslem Spain, and during the Crusades, Western medicine began to develop on its own. Almost ironically, a large shipment of books sent to Alandalus (Moslem Spain) by Byzantine Emperor Alexei Komnenos helped with the development of medicine among the Islamic and Jewish doctors in Spain. The rise of humanism in the West also compensated for the problem of Gnostic dualism, and the awakening of the Western mind to science brought constant developments in medicine to the fore. After the destruction of Constantinople by the Crusaders in the 1200s, Byzantine learning was eclipsed by both Islam and Western Europe as the Eastern Empire expended all of its energies on the struggle for survival and efforts to stave off its political and economic decline. This decline and eventual collapse of the Byzantine Empire did not happen before its medical corpus had been transferred to the Arabs, primarily at Jundishapur, where Nestorian Christians from Constantinople and Edessa had established a school.

2
HISTORICAL SKETCH
The Question of the Site of the Soul and its Impetus to Scientific Medicine and Neurology.

Thou hast set the head as the highest part of the body and endowed it with the senses, which do not impede one another.[10]

Records of the development of medicine go back as far as the Egyptian physician and vizier Imhotep, the "father of pyramid building,"[11] in the reign of Pharaoh Dzhoser, who ruled from about 3000 B.C. Papyrus records from as early as 2000 B.C. contain medical instructions and even prescriptions. In Mesopotamia — the location of Chaldaea and Babylon, regulations dealing with doctors are as old as 1900 B.C.

Since the scope of this paper is limited to the

influence of Orthodox Christian thought on the development of medicine, we cannot digress to these fascinating stories. We will simply note that medicine as we conceive it now began with Hippocrates of Kos (ca.460 B.C.), who instituted careful record keeping and case histories as an aid to transforming medicine into an actual science. We will note, also, that few questions spurred on the philosophy of medicine more than the question of the nature and location of the "hegemonikon," the Prime Centre or soul.

Both philosophers and physicians, as well as many early Christian writers, were interested in the question of the location of the soul in man, although what was meant by a "soul" might not always have been clearly defined.

Early Ideas About the Location of the Soul, Mind and Emotions

It is difficult to actually know what the more ancient writers truly believed about the location of the Prime Centre *(nous: mind/soul/intellect /emotions)* — that is, the dominant control centre of the person. It is doubtful if the earliest speculators had the full range of concepts that developed in later centuries. We speak of the mind, the intellect, soul, spirit and emotions, and when referring to them, do not always mean the same thing from one time to the next.

In the Hebrew Scripture (our "Old Testament"), we are presented with some mention of various organs of the body in this regard. In general, the heart is credited as the locus for the central control of motor responses. It is difficult to say when references to the heart in connection with the Prime Centre (hegemonikon) *(nous: mind/soul/intellect/emotions)* and emotions are clinical, and when they are metaphorical. In the earliest writings, therefore, we have little basis for assuming that they are presenting medical theories.

We do know that the ancient Egyptians thought that the heart was the locus of consciousness. By about 2000 B.C., they were at least aware that motor functions were directed from the brain. Unfortunately, they do not seem to have followed up this valuable clue, although an unnamed military physician did, in about 2000 B.C., make sophisticated notes about it. He noted that injuries to certain parts of the brain resulted in the loss of specific motor functions.

By the fifth century B.C., the Pythagorean philosopher Alkmaeon of Croton,[12] the founder of empirical psychology, had established that the brain was the seat of sensations, and Democritos of Abdera, the Atomist (c.460-360),[13] had correctly asserted that the brain was the location of thoughts, intelligence and the Prime Centre *(nous: mind/soul/intellect/emotions).*[14]

Epicurus, as also the stoics Apollodorus, Chrys-ippus and Protagoras,[15] had asserted that the seat of the *nous (soul/ mind/emotions/personality/spirit)*[16] was in the blood of the pericardium — the blood entering and leaving the heart.

Plato (427-347 B.C.) was a dualist in the

mode of Orphic Gnosticism, to which he belonged. He believed in a radical dichotomy in the nature of man, with the soul and body essentially opposed to each other. Plato taught that, after death, the soul can have knowledge of his "transcendent forms," because it is now pure (being separate and independent of the body). This teaching, expressed in Plato's *Phaedo* is the source of this heresy not only in Latin thought, but also among teachers of error within the Orthodox Church.

This form of dualism, which the Gnostics were fond of, had a negative impact on early medicine. Ironically, Plato's student Aristotle, who refuted this dualism, located the Prime Centre *(nous: mind/ soul/intellect/emotions)* in the heart. In his **Juventate**, Aristotle presents his erroneous reasons for rejecting the brain as the seat of senses and emotions. It is ultimately the Aristotelian Scholastic view of the heart that is used by some to argue against heart transplants. Ironic, too, is the fact that Aristotle became the authority for interpreting the purely metaphorical references to the "heart" in Scripture.

It is difficult to say whether other writers, such as Titus Lucretius Carus were being anything more than poetic in referring to the heart as the place where "fear and terror leap" and "joy gently throbs."[17] The heart certainly responds to the brain's chemistry that generates these impulses, but it initiates nothing. The fact that the brain instructs the heart to respond to stimuli when necessary, and the reaction of the heart is so prominent, sufficiently explains the errors of ancient anatomists and the entrancement of poets.

Tertullian accepted the idea that the site of the soul was in the pericardial blood. The Stoics and others based their theory on animal vivisection, but Tertullian was opposed to such animal experimentation, and, following Aristotle, based his conclusions on figurative scriptural references to the heart with regard to thoughts, feelings and emotions.[18] Actually, Tertullian's belief that the soul was corporeal and had a specific physical site in the body was not advantageous to the advancement of medicine, particularly his acceptance of the idea that the soul/mind/intellect *(nous)* was located in the heart.

It was ultimately the Orthodox Christian concept of man as a psychophysical being, in which neither the soul nor the body alone comprises the person, but the two in unison, which gave direction to their response about the place and nature of the soul. While the philosophers, whom Tertullian so strongly opposed, approached the question from a more esoteric point of view, the Orthodox Christian Church fathers' approach was more pragmatic, as was that of the pagan physicians. Galen's elaboration of the work of the Alexandrians, for example, was influenced by the early Christian Church writers and fathers who advanced theories which interacted with the investigations of non-Christian physicians.

It is clear, then, that the question of the nature and location of the soul became as much a medical and physiological question as a philosophical one. As we shall see, it led to the beginnings of the science of neurology and the proper under-standing of the brain and heart. This direction was taken by those Christians who would research and speculate on the subject, precisely because of the concept of man as a psychophysical being, in which to treat the body was to treat the soul, and to treat the soul was to treat the body. The soul, according to the Orthodox Christian Church fathers, has no form of physical body of its own,[19] but depended on the physical body for its func-tions and senses.[20] This made the treatment of the body as important as the treatment of the soul: physical health was linked to spiritual and mental health.

The Alexandrian (Dogmatist) School

One of the main schools to descend from the great Hippocrates of Kos was that of the "Dogmat-ists" in Alexandria. Perhaps the most significant advances in medical anatomy were made by this school, although they came at a terrible price.

The founder of the Alexandrian school,

Dioclese of Karystos, understood that medical practitioners needed to discover the hidden causes of diseases. By the 400's B.C., the best minds in medical philosophy discounted the notion that demonic influences were the sources of physical illness. In Hellenic society, Hippocrates of Kos had already sounded the final bell for shamanistic

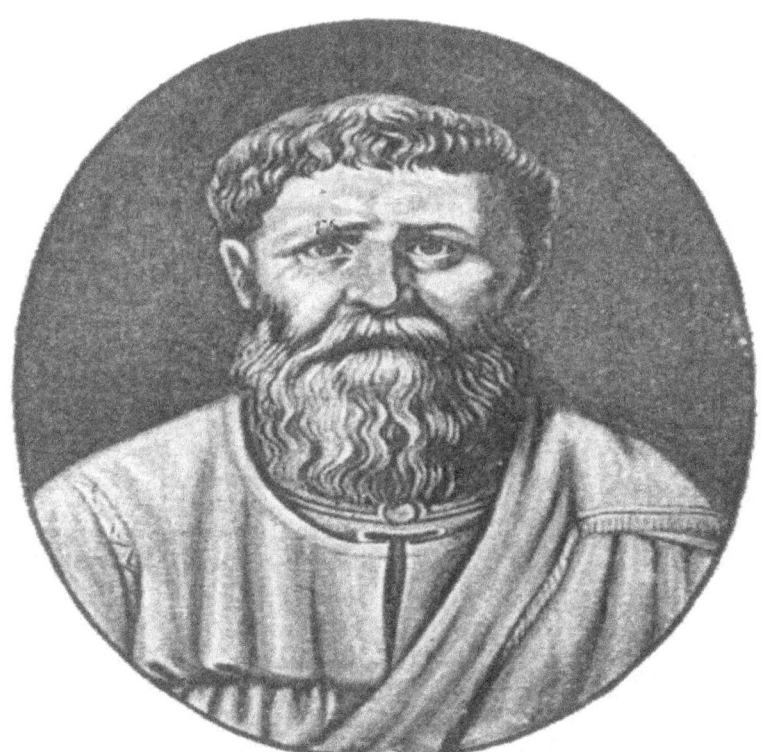

HIPPOCRITES OF KOS

medicine and impelled the philosophy on toward authentic science.

This quest for more accurate knowledge of disease pathology led to some horrendous practices. As mentioned earlier, the Alexandrian School, known as the "Dogmatists," practised vivisection. They often obtained prisoners from the magistrates of the city and literally dissected them while they were still alive. We do not know if the victims were drugged before being dissected, but the Alexandrians justified their practice on the basis of the good that was derived from the experiments. This may not have shocked everyone at the time, considering the liberal use of torture in that era, but is it certainly horrifying. In later times, not only the Christians, but many of the pagan physicians, including Celsus, protested against it. The medical advances of the Dogmatists were, however, impressive

Herophilos and Erasistratos, who worked in the third century B.C. are the most famous members of this school. Herophilos of Chalcedon was a student of Praxagoras of Kos (+ca.340 B.C.), the third leader of the Dogmatist School. He made important definitions of the areas of the brain and asserted that the brain was the seat of intelligence and the organ of the soul.

It was, however, probably his younger contemporary Erasistratos who began to shift attention away from the pericardial membrane, and toward the brain. He held that a combination of the heat generated by the heart and air drawn in produced a substance in the left ventricle of the heart, which he called the "vital spirit." Some of this spirit passed to the brain where it was rarefied and became what was known as the "spirit of the *anima*," a word which, like *nous*, could mean either mind or soul.[21]

Galen of Pergamum

Galen was a physician to the gladiators and the first known practitioner of "sports medicine." He undertook to perfect the work of the Alexandrians. Taking over the idea of the animal or "animating" spirits or "spirit of the *anima*," which he declared to be manufactured in an elaborate network of arteries at the base of the brain, the *rete mirabile* (which, alas, is nonexistent in humans, though found in cattle),[22] he declared that the animal spirit was stored in the ventricles and that its movement from one ventricle to another was controlled by the choroid plexus when the spirit moved between the lateral and third ventricles and by the vermis when it moved between the third and fourth ventricles. According to Galen, however, the soul or mind was in the substance of the brain and not in the ventricles. His reason for this contention was that traumatic lesions of the brain which penetrate to the ventricles could deprive the individual of sensory and motor activities (a fact already known in ancient Egypt), but they were not necessarily immediately fatal as would be expected if the soul resided in the ventricular system.[23]

As Crombie mentions,[24] for Galen, the three principle organs of the body were the liver, which he thought was the font of the blood vessel system, the heart, which combined air from the lungs with blood from the liver, and the brain which is the seat of the nervous system and mental or psychological facilities. The "animal spirit" which Galen thought to be contained in the ventricles of the brain, formed the liaison between the immaterial soul and the material body.

Poseidonius of Byzantium
And Cerebral Localization

The acceptance of cerebral localization was of prime importance to the development of medicine, and this development was largely a result of the questions about the location of the "soul," and the emotions. That Byzantine medical researchers could transfer their attention from the *symbolic* seat of thought and emotions in the heart, to the actual site in the brain is significant.

By the beginning of the third century A.D.,

the ventricular system and the choroid plexus had been identified. Although there was to be no further practical study of the brain for centuries, an associated development, the localization of psychological functions within the cerebral ventricles, was soon to take place. Its exact origins are difficult to determine, but we know that a Byzantine physician Poseidonius (ca.370), had begun the process of brain mapping, and related mental function to particular areas of the brain probably toward the end of the fourth century A.D. His deductions, like those of the ancient Egyptian military physician, may have been based originally on the clinical observations of patients with head injuries. In any event, Poseidonius considered that lesions in the front of the brain interfered with the appreciation of sensation of all kinds, whereas those of the posterior part resulted in a memory defect. Furthermore, he decided that damage to the middle cerebral cavity, that is, our third ventricle, produced a disturbance of reason. Here for the first time, a single mental function was localized in a single cerebral ventricle.[25] This took medical knowledge, and the medical dimension of the question about the soul's location, a great step further in its advancement.

Other Orthodox Christian theorists took up Poseidonius' idea of ventricular localization within his lifetime. Sometime around 400 A.D., Nemesios, Bishop of Emesa, who was well educated in classical medicine and became one of the earliest researchers to map the brain, placed all psychological activities in the cerebral ventricles. He considered each ventricle to be responsible for a specific activity. In his view of the organization of the brain, the anterior (lateral) ventricle, was responsible for the mixing of sensations and for imagination; the middle (third) ventricle, for cogitation and reason; and the posterior (fourth) ventricle, was responsible for memory. Although this follows Galen who established the main faculties of the "sensitive soul," he did not localize them in the ventricles.[26]

The realization that specific areas of the

brain had specific mental and motor functions was of great importance, but without the technical instruments to examine them, no exactness in theory could be established, although considerable strides forward were made. Nemesios schemata or "brain map" remained the standard for centuries.

By the beginning of the fifth century, the shift from the brain substance to the brain ventricles was nearly complete, and support for the contention that the heart was the prime organ, though it survived in philosophy through the medieval period, and in poetry up until our own time, was distinctly less influential as the realization that the heart is a pump with no mental, spiritual or emotional centres and only responds to hormones, etc generated by the brain. This event was of prime importance in the advancement of medical and psychological science. The strongest element in the final development of the ventricular localization theory seems to have been a religious one. Christian fathers and writers considered the soul to be a substance without any form of a body of its own;[27] hence it could not be localized in any corporeal substance, but was joined to the body as light is joined to air. Nevertheless functions of the mind, imagination, reason, and memory could be localized, and most investigators realized that the place to look for them was in the brain, where there were two possible sites, the brain substance and the ventricles. The choice seems to have been decided by those theologians who believed that the spaces of the ventricles provided a more suitable intermediary between the body and the non-corporeal soul than did the solid substance of the brain.[28]

To explain the supposed functioning of the ventricular localization theory, one must understand that it was based on the principle that all thought depended on the perception of sensations. When all types of sensation from the various sense organs were brought together, the *sensus communis* resulted. The *sensus communis* meant, therefore, the mixing of sensations, or "senses in common," but not "common sense" as we think of that term today. When a person began to think, a mixing of the indrawn sensations was believed to occur which in turn produced imagination or fantasy. Since this was the first operation to take place, it was believed to occur in the front of the brain, that is, in the lateral ventricles. The images or fantasies procured in this manner then had to be digested in the action of reasoning or cognition, which occurred in the middle cell or cavity, our third ventricle. Some thoughts were retained for storage, and this process was the memory, which was located in the posterior or fourth ventricle. Thus, the brain function was believed to be a three-stage sequence of imagination, digestion, and retention.[29] The next step was to find appropriate explanations for these processes which would be consistent with the principles of humoural pathology. This difficulty was solved by applying the model of nutrition.

The anterior cell, the lateral ventricles, was declared to be soft and moist since such a climate was believed to facilitate the mixing of sensations and the production of imagination. The next process, thinking or reasoning, was thought to be like the digestion of food which needed heat, and the most appropriate place for it was the warmest, that is, the middle or third ventricle. The posterior or fourth ventricle, the location of the memory, was cool and dry, as these qualities were believed ideal for storage purposes.

In time, a dynamic element was added to the basic doctrine. Galen's idea of valves, the choroid plexus and the vermis, was introduced to the doctrine of ventricular function. They were believed to regulate the flow of animal spirit in the ventricular system. Thought processes, it was believed, could be regulated and the mental responsiveness of an individual was determined by the speed of events in the ventricles. Furthermore, the position of the head could control the valves. For example, throwing the head back while trying to remember was thought to move the vermis, and allow the free passage of spirits from one ventricle to another. If the head were bent forward, however, the vermis would close the passage and concentration would be possible. Only the basic form of the ventricular doctrine has been mentioned here, but since the doctrine dominated all considerations of the brain during the Middle Ages, there were in fact many variants of it. Several dozen of them are to be found as illustrations in medieval manuscripts and early printed books.[30]

There are many other examples of Byzantine medical investigators and writers, but we will mention only three more.

It was the Byzantine physician and medical encyclopedist Oribasios (A.D. 325-403) who made the works of the famous physician Galen of Pergamum accessible to all medical practitioners in the Roman Empire. His massive medical encyclopedia, *The Synopsis*, compiled much of the ancient medical knowledge that was so necessary to the continued development of this science.

Alexander of Tralles (c.A.D. 525-605) was a physician who wrote on pathology, internal medicine and the effects of intestinal parasites. Paul of Aegina contributed his important treatise on surgery, written in about A.D.650.

The Orthodox Christian Doctrine On the Relationship Between Soul and Body

> *Man, with respect to his nature, is most truly said to be neither soul without body, nor, on the other hand, body without soul; but is composed of the union of body and soul into one form of the beautiful.* " (St. Methodios of Olympus).[31]

Man was created both body and soul. The body alone, though it was created first, is not the human being, and though the soul gave life to the body, neither is it alone the human being.[32] Man became a living human being when body and soul were united together.[33] As our holy and God-bearing father Gregory Palamas says:

*When God is said to have made man
according to His image, the word man
means neither the soul by itself nor the
body by itself, but the two together.*[34]

From love, God created the body and in love
He bestowed upon it the soul as the force of life,
that it might dwell in harmony with the body and
function by means of the body, bearing not only
His likeness and image, but man being himself like
a type and image of the life of the Holy Church.
For God created not without wisdom, but that His
love and salvation might be made manifest.

The soul and the body, then, are not two
separate entities; they are together a single
psychophysical whole, mutually serving one
another and mutually dependent upon one another
for life and functions, as our holy father Ephraim
the Syrian says:

*Behold how both the soul and the body
look and attest to one another: even as
the body must have the soul so as to live,*

so must the soul have the body to see and hear.[35]

And St Anastasios of Sinai informs us likewise that:

Accordingly, when the soul is separated from the entire body, it no longer is able to operate, because it operates through the members of the body...[36]

The soul is not the prisoner of the body,[37] rather the two were created and composed together in a mutual life, each one harmoniously deriving functions and qualities of existence from the other.[38] If the soul departs the body, the body dies. And the soul, when separated from the body is no longer able to function in any sensual, psycho-physical manner, as our holy and God-bearing father Justin the Martyr says:

For as in the case of a yoke of oxen, if one or other is loosed from the yoke, neither of them can effect anything, if they be unyoked from their communion... For what is man but the rational animal composed of body and soul? Is the soul by itself man? No; but [only] the soul of a man. Would the body be called man? No; but it is called the body of a man...then neither of these is by itself man, but that which is made up of the two together is called man ...[39]

Thus, the soul and body mutually depend upon, fulfil and provide life and functions to one another. It is sheer carelessness and a great error to misrepresent certain passages of Apostle Paul, using them out of context to establish an idea of a direct conflict between body and soul, and a need for the soul to be liberated from the body. When, for example, the Apostle says, "O wretched man that I am, who will deliver me from the body of this death,"[40] he is referring not to the physical body, but to the power of sin lodged parasitically in the "flesh."[41] To understand the Orthodox Christian anthropology in this respect, one must refer to the Scripture and understand Apostle Paul's teachings, not according to the ideas and conceptions of pagan Greece,[42] which made a sharp distinction between body and soul, but rather to the uniform concepts of the entire Old and New Testament in which "body and soul" denote the whole living person, and not at all independent parts of him. The Manicheans held the contrary view, and St Titus of Bostra, in refuting them, observes:

> When the living body is dissolved by death and we should look upon its dust or its bones, or wish to say something about the soul, we say that these things are of a man, but we do not say that they are the man.[43]

And St Photios the Great, refuting Origenism, concurs:

> The name `man', according to the most truthful and natural expression, applies to neither the soul without [its] body, nor to the body without [its] soul, but to that composition of soul and body made into

a unique form of beauty. But Origen
says that the soul alone is the man, as did
Plato.[44]

In both Old Testament Scripture and general
Hebrew thought, and in New Testament Scripture
and Orthodox Christian thought in general, a
living person is consistently regarded as a compos-
ite entity of body and soul. Death is an unnatural
shattering of this psychophysical entity. As our
holy father St Titus of Bostra says:

But though the soul be immortal [by
grace], yet it is not the person, and so the
Apostle does not consider [death] to differ
in any wise from destruction..."

It was clearly understood in Old Testament
Scripture that that which survived in death maintained a continuity of identity, and, since Christ
had not yet trampled down the bonds of death and
appeared in the state of the reposed ("hades"), it
was conceived of as existing in a state of wordless,
sightless repose. The soul evidently had some con-

sciousness of future destiny, some active hope, and thus it was neither dead nor devoid of some sort of spiritual awareness, by grace.[45]

Old Testament anthropology, like that of the New Testament never conceived of a naturally immortal soul inhabiting a mortal body from which it might be liberated, but always conceived a simple, non-dualistic anthropology of a single, psychophysical organism. An active, intellectual life or functioning of the soul alone could never be conceived in either Old or New Testament thought. For the soul to function, its restoration with the body as the "whole person" would be absolutely necessary.

The sharp conflict between these two concepts: the Scriptural and the Hellenic, was clearly brought forth in the reaction to Paul's sermon to the Greeks, on the resurrection, found at Acts 17:16-34. Apart from the Stoics and a few others, few of the Greeks would have questioned a concept of the soul continuing to exist, and even being rewarded after death, but the idea of a bodily resurrection astounded them. Their astonish-ment was logical. In general, with some exceptions, they conceived that the soul was a prisoner of the body and escaped, or was liberated from the body by death, and that it gained its highest knowledge and awareness only then. Why, therefore, would anyone want to have the soul reunited with the body in a resurrection[46]

By contrast, there is a parable in the Talmud (the Hebrew commentaries on the "Old Testa-ment") which gives a good example of the Old Testament under-standing of the subject. This parable was given to explain the matter to the simple Jewish people. In it we read:

> *There was a ruler who had an orchard.*
> *When he saw that the choice first-fruits*
> *were ripening, he set two watchmen*
> *over the orchard gate. The one was crip-*
> *pled in his legs, and the other was blind.*
> *The cripple, seeing the ripe and choice*
> *first-fruits, submitted to temptation. He*
> *said to the blind man: take me on your*

shoulders, I will guide you, and we will go to the best tree and take of the first-fruits and eat them. This they did. When the ruler came and saw that the choice first-fruits were gone, he questioned the two watchmen. The blind one replied, `Have I eyes that I could see to take the fruit?' The cripple replied, `Have I legs that I could go and get the fruit?' The ruler, perceiving the matter, made the cripple to sit on the shoulder of the blind man, and he judged the two as one. Even so shall the Holy- One, blessed be He, do on the last day. He will cast the soul back into its body, and He will judge the two as one.[47]

The fathers of the Church have taught the same thing, telling us precisely that the soul cannot receive its reward without the body, as St Ambrose of Milan makes clear, saying:

And this is the course and ground of justice, that since the actions of body and soul are common to both (for what the soul has conceived, the body has carried out), each should come into judgment...for it would seem almost inconsistent that...the mind guilty of a fault shared by another should be subjected to penalty, and the flesh, the author of the evil, should enjoy rest: and that that alone should suffer which had not sinned alone, or should attain to glory not having fought alone, with the help of grace?[48]

St Irenae of Lyons is like-minded when he says:

For it is just that in the very same condition in which they (the body and the soul) toiled or were afflicted, being proved in every way by suffering, they should receive the reward of their suffering...[49]

St Titus of Bostra, rebuking the Manicheans, confirms this thought in words quoted by St John the Damascene:

> *For the soul cannot enjoy anything, or possess, or do anything, or suffer, except it be together with the body, being the same as it was created in the beginning, and thus it enjoys that which is proper to it. This state is lost in death through the disobedience of Adam, and again through the obedience of the one Christ, through hope it receives (in the resurrection) again the state of being a person.*[50]

3

THE GOSPEL
FOUNDATIONS

The Healing Ministry of Jesus Christ as the motivation for Orthodox Christian Medicine and the Hospital System in Byzantium.

."..the Sun of Righteousness shall arise with healing in His wings" (Mal.4:2). "And He spoke to them about the kingdom of God, and healed those who had need of healing" (Lk.9:11).

After His baptism, our Lord Jesus Christ had ascended into the wild mountains above Jericho. There, He revealed to us what His kingdom would *not* be. He rejected every manifestation of worldly power and rule, and revealed that the kingdom of God is that uncreated reign of God, manifested wherever the will of God is being done by those who freely accept His rule and place their faith in Him.

When our Saviour came down from the mount of temptation, He straightaway went up to Galilee of the Gentiles and began to proclaim that the Kingdom of God was at hand. How did He demonstrate the presence of the Kingdom of God? By healing people. He announced the Kingdom, and revealed its nature by healing physical, mental and spiritual illness. The entire ministry of Christ, the Gospel of redemption, was a healing ministry, for redemption consists precisely in healing.

> *And Jesus went about...preaching the Gospel of the Kingdom and healing all manner of sickness and disease among the people...and they brought to Him all peoples who were sick with various diseases and torments, and those who were possessed by demons and those that were mentally ill or palsied, and He healed*

them all (Mt. 4:23- 24).

By this, He first of all demonstrates that He has a higher authority, one not of this world, by which He overthrows the things of this world. This authority is not manifested in political power, military might or great wealth; rather it is demonstrated in the exercise of compassionate love, in the liberation of man from the bondage and marks of the fall. In this latter aspect lies a most profound revelation concerning the nature of Christ's mission and the nature of the Holy Church: the Church is a spiritual hospital and redemption is a process of healing.

Orthodox Perspective

In the creation, man was not subject to illnesses of any sort neither of body or mind. The fallen human nature is in a state of disharmony and internal division and chaos because of its separation from communion with God, because of sin (falling short of the mark). The ultimate result of the fallen nature is death, and the ultimate bondage, the fear of death. All these things are results of man's loss of direct citizenship in and communion with the Heavenly Kingdom. Christ came to rescue and restore the human nature which, in Him, was once more perfect, once again united with God. Thus, it is only natural that, since He intended by His life, death and Resurrection to offer the healing of the whole nature of man, He should begin by healing the symptoms and marks of the fall. In this way, Christ brought the consciousness of people to an understanding of the nature of His Kingdom and of His own person. For, having proclaimed, "The kingdom of Heaven is at hand," He immediately begins to overthrow the marks of those things which separate us, our nature, from that Kingdom. Finally, He overthrew the bondage of the fear of death *(Hb.2:15)*, and ultimately even the existence of death will vanish in the full manifestation of His Kingdom *(1Cor.15:26)*. Christ's Kingdom began to be manifested in the healing and transformation of the "inner man" together with the physical man, so that he could be united to the whole body of the Church, now being re-formed in the very midst of the old, corrupted Israel. The Kingdom of God is formed by the liberation of man from the bondage of worldly corruption, and the transformation, and finally the transfiguration of the whole person into a new creature.

Thus the message of mankind's redemption is preached in a manner which also explains the nature of redemption: the healing and restoration of the fallen, universal nature of mankind. The death and Resurrection of Christ makes union with that redeemed nature possible, through union with the perfect Human Nature in Christ. Because Christ redeemed us from bondage to the fear of death (Hb.2:15) with which Satan kept us in thrall, we metaphorically use the expression that "He ransomed us..."

That the message of redemption is a message of healing was made clear by Christ when He healed the paralytic:

..When Jesus saw their faith, He said to the paralytic, Take heart son, thy sins are forgiven. At this, some of the lawyers said in themselves, `this fellow is blaspheming!' Knowing their thoughts, Jesus said, `Why do you harbour evil thoughts in your hearts? Which is easier to say, `Thy sins are forgiven,' or to say `Get up and walk'? But so that you may know that the Son of Man has authority on earth to forgive sins (and he said to the paralytic), `Arise, take up your pallet and go home' (Mt. 9:2-7).

Thus, the whole message of redemption and salvation is one of healing, and this healing is not divided into categories. Christ does not heal only a part of the person, but the whole person: body and soul together as one. These two concepts are of the greatest importance to understanding the relationship between Orthodox Christianity and the development of medicine in the first centuries of our era: Christ's work was not a juridical expedition, but a healing ministry; and this healing pertains to the complete, psychophysical organism that is man — not to a part of that person only, but to the whole person, body and soul as one complete person.

4

THE CHURCH AS
SPIRITUAL HOSPITAL

*When the Roman Empire encountered
the Christian Church, it...was not con-
fronted by simply another religion or
philosophy, but by a well organised society of psychiatric clinics which cured the
happiness-seeking sickness of humanity
and produced normal citizens with self-
less love, dedicated to the radical cure of
social and personal ills. The relationship
between State and Church which developed was exactly parallel to that between
the State and modern medicine. "* (John
Romanides)[51]

Fr John Romanides discusses the Church in
terms of a healing clinic — or rather an associa-

tion of such clinics — in which the spiritual and psychiatric ills of humanity are to be treated. He might also have mentioned that the Orthodox Christian Church, free of the Platonistic and Gnostic influences that plagued the thought of Augustine of Hippo, also became a significant source for the advancement of physical medicine, and generated a profoundly holistic concept of humanity and the healing of humanity. He has touched upon a profound and almost forgotten reality of Orthodox Christianity. We cannot deal here with the important subject of the patristic tradition of psychotherapy, but we will look briefly at how the Orthodox concept of the holistic healing of the psychophysical being of man influenced clinical medicine.

To refer to the Orthodox Church as a spiritual hospital is simply to state the Church's own understanding of itself. A midrash on the parable of the Good Samaritan can offer us an insight into the way early Christians understood the Church. In the parable of the Good Samaritan, one considered to be an "outsider" is the only person with genuine compassion. He dresses the wound of the man who had been beaten, stripped and robbed of all that he had. The "outsider" takes the man to an inn, and provides for him to be kept there until the stranger returns. At that time, this "outsider" will balance all accounts. Let us understand this to mean that Christ has found us spiritually wounded, stripped of our "first image," and robbed of the grace and glory in which we were origially created. He binds our wounds and places us (humanity) in the care of the Church until His Second Coming. The Church, then, is the hospice in which our spiritual wounds are treated and we are, little my little healed and made ready for the

Second Coming of Christ. Indeed, the Church does not send anyone to heaven or to hell, rather it only prepares us for the moment when we will come face to face with the love and glory of Christ our God, as He returns in the fulness of His glory.

As we have noted, when Christ proclaimed that the Kingdom of God was at hand, He demonstrated this with healings of the whole person— physical, spiritual and mental. The Gospel teaches us that the "person" consists, neither in a soul without its body or a body without its soul, rather the person is a union of the two, working together. While the spiritual life of the Church is one of healing the inner person, medicine was considered to be a natural ministry of the Christian faith. This concept had a profound impact on the development and practice of medicine, the hospital and hospice systems in the Orthodox Christian world.

Moreover, the asceticism in Orthodox Christian life, not only that of the monastics, but all the faithful, has always been conceived as part of the healing of the fallen human nature, the healing of the passions. This is at the root of all the periods of fasting and prayer in the Church. Confession, too, is seen as spiritual medication, a door to repentance in which we obtain not only God's forgiveness, but also a reconciliation to a healthy relationship with our own conscience. This healing is spiritual and psychological. Such concepts carried over into the treatment of mentally ill people and the first refuge for the mentally ill based solely on compassion, outside the monasteries, was built at Constantinople.

It was this holistic concept of humanity and a soteriology of healing that inspired the whole movement of Byzantine medicine and healthcare. This is summarised in the words of St Basil the Great:

> *This is foremost in the Saviour's incarnate ekonomia: to gather human nature to itself and to Himself and, having abolished this evil cleavage, to restore the original unity, as the best of physician binds up a body that has been broken in*

many places, using healing ointments.[52]

Redemption and salvation have nothing to do with a human sacrifice of Christ to satisfy God's "justice" and pay a "just death penalty" for mankind. We have been redeemed from the bondage in which Satan holds us by Christ's victory of over death, since "through fear of death, man was all his lifetime held in bondage by him who held the power of death, that is, the devil" (Hb.2:14-15) Christ ransomed us from the power of death, and thus from our bondage to Satan. We are now in the process of our spiritual healing, preparing for our encounter with the visible love and glory of Christ our God.

5

PATRISTIC CONTRIBUTIONS TO MEDICAL SCIENCE.

This is foremost in the Saviour's incarnate ekonomia: to gather human nature to itself and to Himself and, having abolished this evil cleavage, to restore the original unity, as the best of physician binds up a body that has been broken in many places, using healing ointments.[53]

St Basil the Great and the anthropocentric Cosmos

A primary reason that the Cappadocian fathers were able to make contributions to the development of medicine is the fact that they did not disdain secular learning. Indeed, these Church fathers read secular texts in every field of scholarship and utilised elements from this literature for the advancement of Christianity, medicine and social services.

We are interested here in the human-centred universe in the thought and writing of St Basil the Great, and how this concept contributed to the development of the hospital system.

The fundamental purpose in the anthropocentric cosmological ideas of St Basil and those of the early Christian philosopher Clement of Alexandria and his successors was Christian apology, not medicine *per se*. Just as they amended classical dicta in order to accommodate the doctrine of the soul in the example of the formulation of the cerebral ventricular localization theory,[54] Christian apologists strove to use classical learning to sustain other aspects of Christian dogma. One of the most systematic of these undertakings was St Basil the Great's ***Homilies on the Hexaemeron***, a series of nine lectures explaining the text of the opening passages of Genesis where the creation of the world is described.[55]

Designed to uproot and supplant the cosmological tenets of the Greco-Roman world, these exegetic sermons begin with St Basil's acknowledgment that God's creation of the universe is the literal truth. Furthermore, St Basil tells us that the universe was created and exists not for its own sake, but for man's sake. Its purpose is to provide the framework in which each human can and must work out his own destiny. In St Basil's view, since man is the reason for the universe's existence, the study of human structure, functions, and health is in itself of great merit. Thus, St Basil introduced a new idea into the field of cosmology, that the universe can be explained only in terms of man — and this means the complete material/spiritual being of man. The introduction of this anthropocentrism into the field of cosmology coupled with the earlier rejection of Gnostic dualism provided an important impetus for the further study of human sickness and health.

It is extremely important to recognize this

coupling of anthropocentric cosmology with the rejection of that Gnostic dualism which taught that the soul is or has a "subtle body" of its own, and that the soul is essentially the person (like the pagan Egyptian *ka*'). For the Gnostics, the soul was a "divine spark" which was self-subsistent and naturally immortal. It was not at home in this material world, but was rather trapped in the "evil world of matter" (including the human body).[56] St Basil's anthropocentric cosmology was a complete rejection of all ideas of such a dichotomy in the human person and any form of dualism.

The Orthodox Christian doctrine that the soul alone is not the person, nor is the body alone, but only the two in unison make up the person, was important to the development of both medicine and psychiatry. St Basil's awareness that man is a psychophysical being, created by the express intent and will of God made holistic healing a godly pursuit. Anthropocentric cosmology has been increasingly disdained by philosophers in this century. It has, however, reappeared among a number of cosmologists in our own era.

St Gregory of Nyssa

Anthropology, the understanding of "man" is central to theology and to medicine. The Cappadocian fathers were concerned with both. Many writers have suggested that Gregory of Nyssa's teaching on the nature and destiny of man is the crown of this anthropology. His *On the Making of Man* was a primary source for the transmission of Greek medical nomenclature to the West. The unity of soul and body is central to the theme of all Eastern Orthodox anthropology, and had a major impact on incorporating medicine into the Orthodox Christian faith. Gregory of Nyssa's work was written to amplify the anthropocentric cosmology of his brother Basil's *Hexaemeron*. Gregory emphasizes the idea that, since the world was prepared for man's sovereignty, the human body was designed as the ideal repository of both "the mind and the rational soul."[57]

Gregory acquired most of his medical knowledge from Galen, as is clear from his treatise. Like Galen, Gregory was concerned with the meaning and use of things, that is to say, with teleology.[58] The excellence of human hands, Gregory argued, demonstrated the Creator's intention of endowing men with instruments for performing tasks worthy of their god-like minds, while the complex of human vocal organs enabled humans to express their thoughts in the most efficient and effective manner.*** Denying the contentions of others who had localized the soul in the brain or the heart, St Gregory insisted that the rational soul permeated the entire body, vivifying and controlling it.[59]

St Gregory's Theory of Neural Inception

A distinctive element in St Gregory's discussion of the relationship of body and soul is his

advancement of a variant theory of neural inception. Although Galen related that the Alexandrian
anatomist Erasistratus had at one point in his
career traced the motor nerves to the cerebral
meninges, Galen strongly opposed this hypothesis.
St Gregory tells us that certain anatomists believed
the ambient cerebral membranes to be the root of
sensation and motion, and he accepted this thesis.
Although the sources for St Gregory's
breakthrough and comprehensive theory of menin-
geal control over nervous function may have been
influenced by many sources, it is possible that he,
like Celsus, possessed some knowledge of Alexandrian findings not preserved in the extant collection of Galen's theories. In any event, St Gregory's
views concerning the role of the meninges in
nervous function represent a departure from the
traditional view of Galen, and indicates that St
Gregory had read and studied broadly all the
existing medical literature.

St Gregory's treatise *On the Making of Man*
played an important part in transmitting Greek

medical nomenclature and concepts to Latin scholars in the early Middle Ages. Translated into Latin twice before the twelfth century, it, like some of St Basil's works, provided the West with small but important samples of the considerable knowledge contained in Greek medical writings. The patristic writings of Orthodox authors and writings of some Eastern heterodox thinkers, provided a secondary channel by which classical medical terms and ideas were transmitted to the Latin world. Byzantine and earlier Greek medical thought was made available to the Arabs, principally owing to the activity of Eastern Christians. In turn, the Arabs transmitted this learning to the West, via North Africa and Spain. As Byzantium withered after the 13th century, the West ascended in all the sciences.

6

THE GNOSTIC THREAT TO MEDICINE

The Orthodox Christian Church Responds

The fact that Evangelist Luke was a physician, and that he was concerned to record Christ's healing work, had an influence on the later history of medicine that may not be immediately obvious. Its significance becomes clear only if one considers the threats posed to classical, holistic medicine by rivals of the early Christian Church. The chief of these during the second century A.D. was Gnosticism, a general movement divided into many schools or sects. We have discussed the problem of Gnosticism elsewhere,[60] so we will only touch on the most salient aspect of it in relation to our discussion. Though Gnosticism predates Christianity,[61] several schools of Christian Gnosticism developed, others utilized some Christian teachings. Certain Gnostics, especially Marcion,[62] introduced his own version of Christian scripture into their systems and so created "Christian heresies." The threat to medicine from religious sources did not end with the ancient Gnostics. It would appear again in various Christian sects in the 19th and 20th centuries, and is still at work in the 21st century.

During the period of the invasions, the "dark ages" in Western Europe, and the early medieval period, the West was not in a position to pursue any of the sciences to any degree. As plagues followed invasions, a heavy darkness of superstition occupied people's minds. Nevertheless, even after the schism of Rome from the body of the Church, the concepts of charity and healing were strongly entrenched and medical science would eventually be restored and advanced to a role of significance.

The concept of "dualism" refers not only to the idea that both good and evil subsist in God, but also that man is radically divided, with the body and soul being in opposition, or at best in uneasy cooperation with one another. The latter teaching gives the soul a fulness of being completely apart from the body. The former idea, that both good and evil subsist in God, sought a solution to the existence of both good and evil which sometimes resulted in the theory of two separate gods involved in creation and redemption. The creation of matter was considered to be the work of the evil side of God, or of the evil demi-god.

The Gnostic teacher Marcion, for example, believed that the writings of Apostle Paul provided a basis for the incorporation into Christianity of Gnostic dualism and a unique ascetic theology aimed against the body. Marcion, like other Gnostic teachers, felt that this dualistic concept was necessary for any explanation of the presence of evil in the world. They gave a strained interpretation to Apostle Paul's words to try to demonstrate a conflict between the human body and the soul. Marcion distinguished between two Gods: the God of the Old Testament, orderer of a matter which he had not created, which was the source of evil in the world, and the God of the New Testament who had remained unknown to men until Jesus Christ had come to reveal him. Unlike the Old Testament God of the Jews who was a judge, this new god, or foreign god, was all goodness.[63] In Gnostic systems, this new God, Jesus, came to liberate the "divine spark" or soul, which was a pure spirit with a subtle body, from the prison of the body — vile matter. The destruction of the body by illness and disease was a positive process, and medical science was not necessarily a good thing. Actually, a number of the Gnostic leaders advocated the destruction of classical medical texts, and only through the efforts of Orthodox Christian writers were these texts saved.[64]

The primary form of this heretical dualism in our own time, within the Orthodox Church, is the "aerial toll house" heresy.

The Church Responds

We will turn to St Irenae of Lyons (125-203) for a summary of the Orthodox response to Gnosticism. He is thoroughly representative of the Orthodox Church fathers in this regard, and he directed his entire writing to the refutation of Gnostic doctrines.

St Irenae teaches that the world was created not out of ignorance or malevolence (as many of the Gnostics thought), but through the love and generosity of its Creator. Like the rest of creation, man had been made good. He was not perfect, being created finite and limited, but was, as it were, an infant in the garden, needing to grow and develop to his ultimate maturity — a parent nurturing a beloved child might readily understand the relationship between God and the first humans. This is an idea profoundly expressed in Orthodoxy iconology, which presents us with a true foundation of morality. Why does the Apostle tell us that

Christ is the express image of the Father *(Col.1: 15; 2Cor. 4:4)*? Because Christ, being truly God, has been incarnate in our form in order to restore in us that image in which man was first created, and restart us on that struggle to full maturity in God's image. Mankind was created in the image of God and is now assigned the task to grow in the likeness of Christ. Christ *healed* and our task is *to become healed*.

Most important to the development of medicine, Saint Irenae (as with all the Church Fathers) consistently opposed the dualistic idea that man's body, being formed of matter, was therefore inferior to his spiritual nature. He maintained that man is essentially a living, rational being whose entire make-up was composed of two essentials, body and soul, and that only soul and body together can be considered the "person."[65]

Thus, St Irenae disassociated the Orthodox Christian faith from every form of Gnostic dualism with its notion that asceticism is a flight *from* life, rather than an *ascent into* life. Gnostic hatred of the body as being intrinsically evil expressed itself in many and variant excesses. Some Gnostics became libertines in order to wear the body out, and hence to free man's spirit sooner from it.[66] Physicians and all those who sought to minister to the body were abhorrent to them. Marcion even prepared an expurgated version of certain sections of the New Testament in which he deleted Paul's reference to Luke as the beloved physician in his letter to the Colossians *(4:14)*.

The Orthodox Christian vision of life in the world does possess a special asceticism which was exciting and exhilarating even to some of the pagan philosophers. It made evil intelligible and good pure, with no blurred lines between the two. Emphasizing the moral responsibility of man, it was very appealing. Moreover, the early Christian ascetical approach did not replace sound theology, but gave a visible, vivid spiritual life to this theology. The Orthodox Christian ascetic does not struggle to become "liberated from life," but rather struggles to become *present to life*. Galen, who respected Christians, but questioned the source of their beliefs, had the following to say of them:

> "So in our own times we see people who are called Christians, and who have created their beliefs from parables. Their outlook corresponds to that of the true philosopher for they despise death, as we have seen before our very eyes.... There are among them both men and women who remain sexually abstinent their entire lives, and there are those who have achieved such a degree of self-control that they are equal to any philosopher."[67]

Galen who was a surgeon to gladiators, thus confirmed and marvelled at the ascetic tendencies of the early Christians. In another of his writings, he asserted that the Christians should be considered as adherents to a *medical* sect.[68] In the second century A.D., therefore, Christianity, as Irenae realized, was at a turning point. Had he and other early apologists not resisted and even combatted the lure of the Gnostics and of the mystery cults toward ascetic theologies, the ideals as well as the texts containing classical medicine's literary treasures would very likely have been destroyed. The interests in and respect for the material aspects of man's nature which Luke the physician exemplified, and the Orthodox Church fathers defended, therefore played a large role in the preservation of classical medical literature.

The early Christian Church provided an important "safety valve" for the dynamic and powerful Gnostic inclinations of the first several centuries of our era. This safety valve was monasticism. The early monasteries were able to absorb and channel Gnostic tendencies into spiritual struggle. Gnostic dualism was often expressed in the form of metaphor and parable in early ascetic writings. Lacking a knowledge of the way the brain and the body function, the movement of the passions were often ascribed to physical organs of the body without reference to the mind. Where Apostle Paul speaks negatively of the "flesh," he is speaking of the presence of sin lodged parasitically in the person, and not disparaging the body. To place a conscious sinfulness in the organs of the body is sheer superstition and ignorance and, as we shall see, is radically contrary to the teachings of the holy fathers. Unfortunately, through Gnostic tendencies in some monasticism, dualistic Gnostic errors would become entrenched in some of the Paterikons and would lead Gnostics of later times, including our own, to posit an "ascetic theology," which in so many ways opposes the divine theology of the holy fathers, and is laced with Gnostic ideology. Nevertheless, the effectiveness of this "shock absorber" (monasticism) may be seen in the fact that the Orthodox Church has always advocated married priest in the parishes, while the Latins, more deeply influenced by Gnosticism and Augustinianism, forbade clergy to marry — on essentially Gnostic grounds. The development of medicine and medical ideology in the East may also be seen as a result of this "filter." The formation of Gnostic dualism posed the greatest threat to the development of medicine; why would one develop treatments for bodily ills if the destruction of the body was the liberation of the soul? Let us also note that several of the monastic communities built and operated well staffed and well organised hospitals in Byzantium, as some monasteries in Romania and elsewhere are doing today with medical clinics.

Ignorance of the function of the brain and the nervous system had a great deal to do with the entrenchment of Gnostic concepts and ideas in so much of the ascetic literature in the East, but these ideas did not impede medical experimentation and the preservation of ancient medical texts.

We will not give more attention to this particular problem at this point, but it is necessary to establish the fact that the impetus for the development of medicine in the Byzantine Orthodox world was the image of Christ as the Great Physician, and the holistic concept of the human person. It is notable also, that medicine flourished more strongly in the East because members of noble and wealthier families in Byzantium became medical doctors while in the West, for a few centuries, medicine was a "lower class" profession.

7

THE FOUNDATIONS OF CLINICAL, HOSPITAL AND PSYCHIATRIC CARE

*"For I was hungry and you gave
me food; I was thirsty and you gave me
drink; I was a stranger and you made
me welcome; naked and you clothed me,
sick and you visited me, in prison and
you came to see me" (Mt.25:35-37).*

The Saints and the Medical Tradition

The development of hospital based medical care
began long before Constantinople was built as
a Christian city. The concept of medicine and
health care as a natural Christian ministry began
quite early in Apostolic times and appears to have

been inaugurated by women. While the order of holy unmercenary physicians became the main representatives of this ministry, the medical ministry began with the proto-monastic women's groups and communities. He orders of widows and virgins, which would eventually develop into monasticism, had primary rolls in both charity and medicine.

It may have been the Gospel according to Luke which inspired much of this movement. Evangelist Luke the "beloved physician" was a leading figure in the early Orthodox Catholic Christian Church. Following the gospel of Jesus Christ, salvation has been understood as a process of healing, so it followed logically that with the healing of the fallen human nature, physical healing must be a manifestation of that process. This became a vital aspect of early Christian life.

"The Beloved Physician"
Luke's Gospel

It has become a commonplace of for critics to suggest doubts about the authorship of Luke's Gospel and the Book of Acts. Such doubts are, however, clearly unfounded. The evidence is conclusive that both treatises were written by a physician, and Luke was "the beloved physician" (*Col. 4:14*) who wrote them. Both books demonstrate a knowledge of medicine and in both there are clear signs of medical diction.

It is Luke's Gospel that gives us a clear picture of Christ as the Divine physician, and redemption as a healing process. The reign ("kingdom") of God is proclaimed through the healing of the divisions and wounds in the fallen human nature. The human person is treated as a "whole being," as body and soul together, with no hint of any enmity between the two. Christ's activity as the healer of body and soul is accentuated in the Luke's Gospel where a distinction is clearly made between healing the body of organic illness, and exorcising demons, both mental and spiritual.[69] The symbolism of God as a physician is carried still further in the concluding passages of Luke's *Acts of the Apostles*, where Paul illuminates the book's dominant note by paraphrasing God's proclamation to Isaiah *(6:9-10)* that His healing activity will henceforth be directed no longer exclusively to the Jews but also to the Gentiles *(Acts 28:25-28)*. Salvation is directly linked to healing in this passage.

The distinctive character that Luke, as a physician contributed to the New Testament by his writings is well established and has been discussed by many writers. We will add nothing new, but only invite your attention to what has already been expressed many times.

One might suggest that Luke was called to be an evangelist, as well as a scribe for Apostle Paul, because he was best equipped to understand the healing ministry of Christ.

Apostle Paul tells us directly that Luke was a physician. Passages from Luke's writings containing elements of his scientific knowledge and awareness of the principles of medical diagnosis have been examined by many qualified writers, and scholars have identified places in Luke's writings where language shaded with medical phraseology has been used. Where Luke speaks as an eye witness to an event, he employs not only medical diction, but medical metaphors.[70] Apostle Luke was, therefore, well equipped to establish the concept of the healing process of redemption and demonstrates that healing and redemption pertain to the whole psychophysical being that is man.

8

THE MOTHERS OF
MODERN MEDICINE

There were two sometimes competing medical concepts in the first century of our aeon. The concepts of Hippocrates of Kos advocated a scientific basis for medicine, while the Asclepian[71] system was primarily psychosomatic and oriented toward magic. Hippocrates introduced, or one should say, expanded on, the keeping of medical records and case studies. Many of his followers made important discoveries in medicine and health care.

It must be said that some of the followers of the Asclepian method did reject, the idea of magic in medicine though it still remained tied to amulets, religious formulas and pilgrimages. Some of their psychosomatic approaches were fascinating and often produced good results. There is a positive side to the enhancement of healing through psychological methods and the use of rituals to obtain a placebo effect. However, without the scientific approach and a careful development of pharmacology, the processes could not advance and provide a basis for the development of modern medicine. Within the Orthodox Church, the movement toward a sound, scientific medicine was inaugurated among the earliest Christians. Among these were disciples of the School of Hippocrates and first among them were two often forgotten women.

Tarsus was not only an important metropolis, it was also an imperial city. It was here that Cleopatra came when she wanted to meet Mark Antony. To be born a citizen of Tarsus was to inherit the coveted Roman citizenship.

As a major cutlural centre, Tarsus attracted representatives of every philosophical school. Each school set up its own "academy" and attracted students. Two cousins of Apostle Paul were attracted to the disciples of Hippocrates of Kos and studied medicine with them.

Philonella and Zenaida were sisters of Jason, Paul's cousin who was to become the first bishop of Tarsus. They had become Christians very early, and perhaps even before Apostle Paul. The two sisters had been deeply moved by the example of Christ's life and his teaching. They understood that salvation is a healing process, and that Christ had healed the body together with the soul. Being disciples of Hippocrates' school they were interested in a more scientific approach to medicine and continued the efforts to free medicine from magic and superstition. Their efforts were to have an important impact on the development of the hospital system in Byzantium, and on the formation of modern medicine.

Other great women of the early church made important contributions also. The physical foundations of medical clinics and ultimately, the development of hospital centred medicine, was laid down by Hermione, the daughter of Philip the Deacon (Acts ch.6), the two saints Melanie and

Paul of Palestine. Hermione founded the Xenodo-khia system of shelters, with basic medical care, for strangers who were travelling. The two Melanies, grandmother and granddaughter, (5th century), who were wealthy Romans, established medical clinics and expanded Hermione's work in Palestine. Paula of Palestine (+ AD 404) carried this work to a new level and some of these institutions were of such quality that they could be expanded into small hospitals.

9

DEVELOPMENT OF THE BYZANTINE HOSPITAL SYSTEM

The foundation of the concept of medicine as a ministry of the Church lies in the healing ministry of Christ Jesus. As we have noted, Christ was not manifested on earth for the purpose of a juridical expedition, but rather to reveal the co-suffering love of God with mankind and demonstrate that the Kingdom of Heaven was revealed in healing. The elements of the fallen human nature were made whole again in the man Jesus, and united once more with God in the person of Christ Jesus, Who was Himself both perfect God and perfect man. While He healed people of physical ills, and tied this healing together with the revelation of the Kingdom, at the same time He healed both psychiatric[72] and spiritual illnesses. By His death and resurrection, He also healed the fall of mankind by conquering the power of death. The ultimate process of healing the whole person is called "theosis."

The importance of those acts of mercy mentioned in Matthew's Gospel *(Mt.25:35-37)*, in providing the scriptural impetus for the development of the medical movement and the development of the hospital system, is amply demonstrated by the fact that these acts were depicted iconographically or in other forms of art both inside or outside most hospitals and other charitable institutions funded and supported by both the Church, wealthy patrons and the State in early times. From the beginning of Christian history, therefore, care for the sick was deemed a responsibility of not only individual Christians, but of the whole Church body,[73] and the Christian state itself.

The administration of charitable acts in the early Church was first delegated to the office of the deacon. The office of the deacon was created with to the seven men appointed by the apostles to help serve the Christian community, though the *title* of deacon is first mentioned in Paul's Epistle to the Philippians.[74] Within the first century of Christianity, however, deacons, that is men and women set aside for special service to the Church, became a permanent institution, and special qualifications were laid down for those who held this office, though their functions varied at different times and in different places.[75]

Initially, the deacons were helpers to the bishops (later, also to the priests) and, in a general way, to the congregation also. As the Church developed into an organized body, the deacons became more specifically the direct ministers of the bishop, and their duties included visitation of the sick and ministering to them with the best medical knowledge of the say, distribution of alms, and care for widows and orphan. By the third century, Rome was divided into districts, called deaconries, which were administered by deacons who were immediately responsible to the bishop. In the sixth century, Pope Gregory I reorganized the system, dividing the districts into seven ecclesiastical regions and thirty parishes. Though the parishes were in the charge of priests, the regions were divisions, each headed by a deacon.

The deacons, headed by an archdeacon, were assigned the duty of caring for the poor, widows, orphans and elderly of their districts. Under the guidance of the bishop, they drew up lists of those entitled to draw relief. In Rome, each district had a hospice or an office for alms, of which the deacon, assisted by a steward, was in charge. In Constantinople and the rest of the East, actual hospitals were developed. In addition to the medical care of the ill, in these hospitals food was distributed, meals served, the sick and poor maintained, and orphan and foundling children housed.

Contributions of the Saints
The Holy Unmercenary Physicians

All medicine is *psychosomatic.* In a literal sense, this word means the same as *psychophysical,* and should not carry the almost pejorative connotation that has been attached to it in later times. Psychosomatic medicine utilizes all the weapons available for the treatment of any form of illness. Medication, whether chemical or natural, combined with both faith and a will to be well may all work together in the healing of the human organism, because the person consists in soul, body, mind and spirit, however one perceives the bond of these spiritual, physical and psychological elements. Treating the whole person is far more effective than treating a series of symptoms or simply attempting to exterminate a variety of microbe.

A strong tradition in the Orthodox Christian world was that of the Holy Unmercenary physicians. This category of saint was made up of trained physicians who, being Christian, added not only the holistic dimension to their practice, but treated the poor and disadvantaged without charge for their services. They combined clinical medicine with prayer, never disdaining pharmaceuticals or traditional medical practices.

Among the pioneers of structural medical care in the unmercenary tradition was Hermione, a daughter of Philip the Deacon (Acts chapter 6) whom we mentioned earlier. She was born in Caesarea of Palestine early in the first century. Joined by her sister Eukhidia, Saint Hermione bought a house and founded a medical clinic devoted to the treatment of the poor and the homeless. Rooms were added for poor travellers who were ill. In this way, Hermione started the tradition of Christian hospital-hostels or "xeno-dokhia", which would become so much a part of the function of the early Orthodox Christian dioceses.

While the most famous of these unmercen-ary physicians are Sts Cosmas and Damian, St

Panteleimon and Sts Cyrus and John, all of whom were martyred in the 200's, it was St Samson "the Hospitable" who laid the foundation for the concept of the modern hospital. In Constantinople where, in Justinian's time, an authentic medicare system was in operation, Emperor Justinian commissioned St Samson to create a model hospital. The saint built on the concept of a hospital based on the *xenodokheion* system.[76]

While the origins of modern professional care of the sick may be sought in the history and development of the deacon's office as the overseer and dispenser of Christian charity, the inception of the charitable institutions from which our hospitals evolved may be traced to the *xenodokheion*, a hospice originally designed to receive poor and sick pilgrims. The foundation of the *xenodokheion* as an important and necessary institution in the Christian community was firmly established by A.D. 325.[77] Although the requirement does not appear in the Canons of the First Ecumenical Council, it appears to have been discussed and agreed on at this council, that, in every Christian city, a place be reserved for the reception and care of poor and sick pilgrims.

The requirement clearly responded to a deeply held sense of Christ's injunctions, as it was put into effect virtually immediately. In less than a generation, St Basil the Great, as bishop of Caesarea, established an enormous *xenodokheion* just beyond the limits of his episcopal city. Surrounded by walls, the establishment included dwelling houses, a church, a hospital for the sick, a separate sanitorium for lepers, a hospice for travellers, and a staff of doctors, nurses and artisans. This *Basiliad*, as it was called, was erected on such a vast scale that it was referred to as an entirely new city.[78] Its success, and that of comparable institutions, can be judged by the lament expressed by Emperor Julian the Apostate (361-363 A.D.). Julian sought to return the empire to the paganism of earlier times, but despaired of his chances of such a victory over a faith which conferred such remarkable and tangible health benefits on mankind.[79]

We find the building of hostels, clinics and shelters for both medical and charitable purposes in the lives of many saints in the Orthodox Church, among them St Paula of Palestine and the two Sts Melanie.[80] There was a deep consciousness of holistic healing, which naturally enough, centred on the spiritual aspect of all illnesses, and the ultimate healing of the fallen human nature itself. All of these hospice and clinic developments represented an accumulation of knowledge and experience that led to the development of the modern hospital and hospital based medical care in the Byzantine Empire.

Palliative care hospices were established and maintained in Western Europe also, with the same compassion and care as in the East, but modern hospitals and hospital based medical care would not appear there until centuries later.

How complete these hospitals in Byzantium were can be seen from the details we have about the ones built by Emperor Alexei Komnenos (1169-1183) and his father John II (1087-1143). The hospitals had careful planning for heating, ventelation, lighting, toilet facilities. There was a regulated schedule for changing and laundering sheets. The hospitals had a nutritionist who planned the vegetarian diet provided for the patients. An interesting feature of the health care system was the public baths (most middle and lower class homes did not have baths in the ancient world). Bathing regularly was considered to be necessary for good health. Baths open to the public were found in hosptals and hospices and there were special "women only" days. Public baths had been closed in Western Europe by the religious authorities who felt that they were indecent. One is reminded of the Byzantine princess Theophano. She was married to the German king, and had become unpopular in Germany because she bathed daily and ate with a fork rather than her fingers.

John II had built his hospital in conjunction with the Monastery of the Pantokrator. He provided for faculties devoted to advancing the medical sciences.

10

Cross Fertilization
of Medical Concepts

Preservation of Works of Galen[81] and Celsus[82]

T he Byzantine Empire was in an ideal
geographical location to experience a cross
fertilization of medical ideas from both
Persian, Arabic and Hindi[83] sources. It is not clear
to what degree such knowledge existed in each of
these civilisations. Certainly, the older Hindi and
Persian societies would have been more advanced
than the Arabic in the early centuries. It is also not
clear how much of the then existing corpus of
medical concepts came from which source. What
is known is that the survival of the medical works
of both Galen (A.D.130-200) and Celsus (1st
Century A.D.) substantiate our observation that
the great medical works of antiquity owe their

survival to the anti-Gnosticism of ancient Orthodox Christians. Helpful, too, was the attitude of
the great Church fathers that pagan learning was
not to be feared, but to be studied and built upon.

Since Galen lived a century and a half after
Celsus, and as his authority was well established in
Greek culture, we shall examine the Christian
impact on the survival of his writings later. Celsus,
on the other hand, wrote in Latin, and in very
good Latin.

Celsus compiled his compendium of knowledge titled *Artes*[84] during the reign of Tiberius,
(A.D.14-37). While this work dealt with agriculture, military science, rhetoric, jurisprudence,
philosophy and medicine, only the section on
medicine is still extant. We know of the other
portions of this vast encyclopedia only from
references in other writings. Columella,[85] for
example, quoted Celsus' treatise on agriculture, and
Quintilian[86] criticised Celsus' remarks on
rhetoric,[87] but most of our knowledge of the non-
medical sections of the compendium, comes from

the lengthy apologetical work, *Contra Celsus*,[88] composed by the early Christian philosopher Origen (185-254).

Unlike Galen, who seems on the whole to have been a sympathetic observer of the Christian movement and who admired, as we have seen, the virtues of courage and self-control he saw exhibited by the followers of Christ, Celsus viewed the Christian attitude toward life in this world more critically. He believed Christianity to be basically inimical to science, and compared Christians to uneducated rustics or children who flee from physicians believing knowledge of natural phenomena to be intrinsically evil.[89] This line of argument on the part of Celsus is significant to our present subject because it demonstrates that already in his time, there were two streams developing within Christianity, one Orthodox and one Gnostic, which would give shape to the Latin West. Celsus was more familiar with the Latin developments which were more affected by Gnosticism and neo-Platonism (later, by Aristotelianism). He may, therefore, have even confused Christianity with the Gnostics who appropriated the name of the Christians, and who actually did have the negative dispositions that he criticised.

Origen's goal in his *Contra Celsus* was to answer each of Celsus' objections to Christianity. In order to oppose Celsus' views, Origen cited, and thus preserved, them. Celsus' anti-Christian stance ultimately made his writings unpopular, and after Christianity became accepted within the Roman Empire, copies of the encyclopedia of Celsus, with the exception of the medical section, were virtually all destroyed.[90] The medical section was preserved undoubtedly because the Orthodox Christians found it important and useful.[91]

Though rejecting the arguments Celsus advanced to oppose Christianity, Church writers found they could concur with the moral position he had adopted concerning the ethics of human experimentation. Celsus, as a medical encyclopedist (rather than a physician), related in his account of medical history that Herophilus and Erasistratus, the renowned anatomical investigators who worked at Alexandria during the third century, B.C. conducted anatomical dissections of *living humans.* Celsus, while condemning the procedure, reported that a group of medical practitioners, the Dogmatists, had justified human vivisection on the grounds that the good derived from such practices outweighed the evil of the action.[92]

Celsus' disapproval of human vivisection was echoed by Christian writers such as Tertullian,[93] one of the most influential Western Christian writers of the second century. In general, Tertullian always opposed the Gnostics as well as any kind of philosophical thinking in matters of faith. Nevertheless, he adopted some of the errors of the Gnostics himself.[94] While Tertullian's rigidity eventually led him to become a heretic, he began as an Orthodox Christian and his writings reveal for us the deep respect early Christians had for medicine.

Opposed to most pagan learning, Tertullian coined his famous aphorism, "the philosophers are the patriarchs of heretics" to warn against the danger he believed Christians faced if subjected to a traditional classical education.[95] Nevertheless, his reading of classical medical texts supplied Tertullian with most of his material for the discussion in his *Treatise on the Soul*, chapter 15, on the soul's site in the human body.[96] Philosophers and physicians had long argued over whether the soul had a corporeal site, and if so where it was located. Tertullian tells us Plato claimed its seat was in the occipital section of the head, the primary organ; Hippocrates placed it in the brain, while Herophilus assigned it to the base of the brain; Strato and Erasistratus to the cerebral meninges; and Strato the physicist to the frontal region between the eyebrows.[97]

11
The Transfer of the Orthodox Christian Medical ˙Concepts to the Islamic World.

In 428, the Syrian bishop Nestorius was conse-crated Patriarch of Constantinople. Nestorius ended up falling into serious heresy and was sent into exile.[98]

Despite Nestorius' condemnation, a number of Syrian Christians accepted his teachings and in consequence were forced to emigrate eastward, principally to Edessa where a Christian school of medicine had long flourished. After this educational centre was closed by order of the Emperor Zeno in 489, Nestorians took refuge in Persia whence they carried their doctrines throughout the entire length of Asia. They also took with them the Byzantine corpus of the knowledge of classical and Christian medicine, and hence the Nestorians became significant in the history of medicine by providing, for many centuries, one of the most important links between Byzantine thought and the Middle and Far East.

The medical school at Edessa was succeeded by the schools of Nisibis in Mesopotamia, and Jundishapur in Southern Persia which reached its greatest prosperity during the middle of the sixth century. A great clearinghouse for the exchange of philosophic and scientific ideas, Jundishapur soon became a centre where Greek medical works were translated into Syriac, Persian and, after the Moslem conquest, Arabic. The translating activity at Jundishapur gradually became more and more important until in the ninth century the Caliph, Al-Ma'mun, summoned the translators to Baghdad where he established a school for rendering Greek scientific texts.[99]

The dominating figure of this intellectual

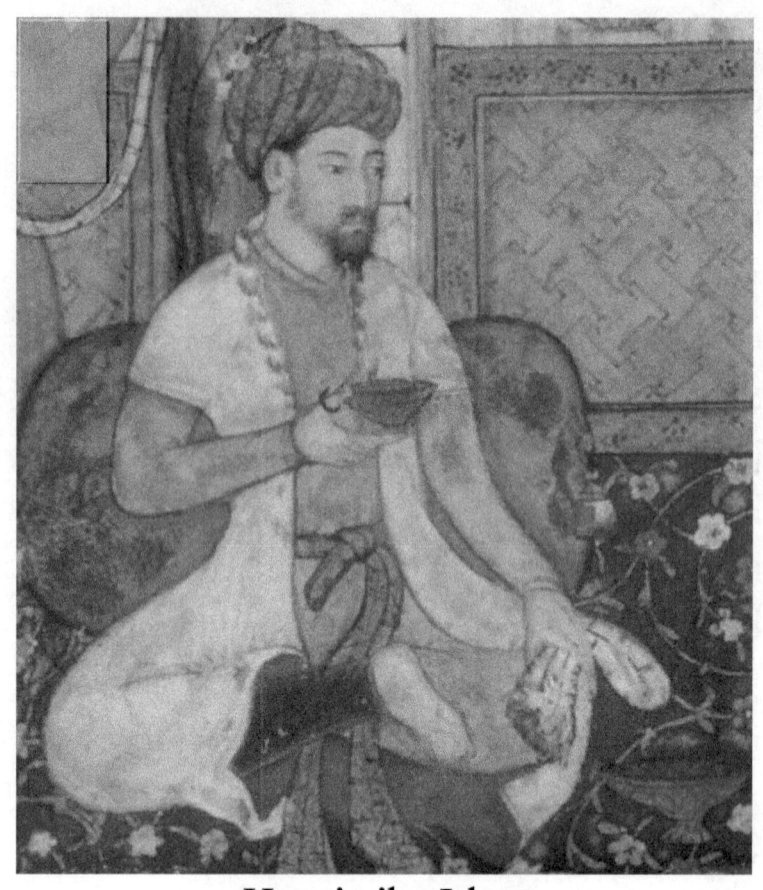

Hunain ibn Ishaq

centre was Hunain ibn Ishaq, a Nestorian Chris
tian, who worked first at Jundishapur and then at
Baghdad where he died in 877. A physician and a
brilliant, productive scholar, Hunain was appointed first director of the translating school at

Baghdad. In addition to his administrative duties, Hunain completed ninety-five Syriac and thirty-nine Arabic versions of authentic, supposed authentic, and spurious Galenic writings. More proficient in Greek and Syriac than in Arabic, he was assisted in his later years by his son, Ishaq, and his nephew, Hubaysh ibn-al-Hasan.[100]

Undoubtedly the greatest medical scholar of the ninth century, Hunain and his followers provided the basis for the golden age of Islamic medicine by bringing the Byzantine corpus and tradition of medical knowledge and practice into the Eastern languages. By 900 A.D., most important Greek medical works were available in good Arabic translations. Hunain's principal interest was the collection of works ascribed to Galen, and his particular viewpoint dominated subsequent Islamic medical thought. The hegemony that Galen's works exerted over the medical thinking of the Moslem as well as of the Western world until well into the sixteenth century is attributable in large part to Hunain's authority and influence.[101]

12
Conclusion

While the writings of patristic authors, with their preservation of the works of earlier medical philosophers and practitioners such as Galen, and the versions rendered by the Nestorian translators set the course for the subsequent growth of medical knowledge, the greatest Christian impact on the care and healing of the sick resulted from the Christian sponsorship of charitable institutions. While these were founded in response to Christ's injunction toward acts of mercy and love found in Matthew's Gospel, cited above, a greater impetus was given to this process by the awareness that the Church itself was a spiritual hospital, and that the real essence of redemption is healing — the healing of the fallen human nature.

Orthodox Christianity profoundly affected medicine and its ancillary disciplines. Classical medicine survived the civilization that produced it largely because of its acceptance by the Orthodox Christian apologists, and their willingness to meld it into the framework of patristic thought. Christian commentators and translators also played a vital role in preserving and disseminating classical medical con-cepts, and owing to their activities, Greek medical writings were read by a much larger audience than their authors could ever have imagined. Orthodox Christianity's most important influence on medical thought and practice, however, was its fundamental gospel of co-suffering love and healing, which re-sulted in sponsoring an individual as well as a corporate concern for the sick and for all human suffering. As Julian the Apostate noted, this was one of Christianity's greatest strengths, and was un-doubtedly the one which exerted its most enduring impact on the subsequent history of the healing arts. I suggest that it also had much to do with the triumph of Christianity over pagan Rome and over Julian's efforts to restore that paganism.

ENDNOTES:

1. Rahner, Karl. *Theological Dictionary*, Herder, Freiberg, 1961. See Khrapovitsky, Metropolitan Antony, "Moral Idea of the Dogma of Redemption," in *The Moral Idea of the Main Dogmas of the Faith*, Synaxis Press, Dewdney, B.C., 1984. Rahner, it must be noted, is not so much drawing a conclusion in the passage quoted, rather he is attempting (vainly) to convince us that there were two separate streams of patristic tradition, both equally valid, both merely stressing certain aspects of a common tradition. His comparison in the cited passage is valid, the idea he has behind it is not.

2. Ironically, one or two of the holy fathers, in refuting certain of the Gnostics, also used the term "subtle body" in relationship to the soul. However, the fathers were using this term to refute the teaching of certain Gnostics that the soul was a "pure spirit" like God. Unlike the Gnostics who were attempting to assert that the soul is the actual person and, having a subtle body, does not need the physical body, the holy fathers used the expression "subtle body" simply to assert that the soul is not a pure spirit like God, but belongs to the realm of the created, material order. For the Gnostic, the term "subtle body" was intended to teach a total self sufficiency of the soul, while for the holy fathers, it was used to assert that the soul is created and not a pure, eternal spirit like God Himself.

3. Rene Descartes (1596-1650). see Damasio, Antonio, *Descartes's Error*, (Grosset/Putnam, N.Y., 1994). Interestingly, Rene Descartes's radical dualism was opposed by his student Princess Elizabeth of Palatine.

4. There is no "‑‑‑‑‑‑‑‑‑" in Orthodox Christian doctrine.

5. see *The Soul, The Body and Death*, (Synaxis Press, 1996) chapter 11

6. *Healing in the History of Christianity* (Oxford University Press, New York, 2005) p.75

7. As the late theologian John Romanides frequently said in his lectures, "The development and practice of unselfish love is the only means for defeating the power of Satan."

8. *The Birth of the Hospital in the Byzantine Empire* (Johns Hopkins, Baltimore, 1997) p.97 (Cited in Porterfield).

9. *Historical Trends and Doctrinal Themes* (Fordham, New York, 1975),p.75 (Cited in Porterfield).

10. From the prayer of the tonsure in the Baptism Service.

11. Imhotep designed and supervised the building of the "step pyramid" for Pharaoh Dzhosher, the first of the pyramids. Completed in appromiately 2700 B.C., it appears to have been based on the structure of the ziggurats in Chaldea.

12. Alkmaeon of Croton (c.500 B.C.) was a student of the mystic mathematician Pythagoras. He discerned that the brain was the seat of sensations and thought and was, perhaps, the first to distinguish between veins and arteries and mention the visual connection between the eyes and the brain. He performed the first recorded dissections of humans (although not vivisection) and attempted to define the nature of disease.

13. The originator of the atomist theory, Democritus' ideas were influential in the Alexandrian School, but fell into disfavour until nearly the 19th century.

14. We sometimes use the term *"hegemonikon"* rather than soul, mind, intellect, etc because we are referring to the governing faculty of all those. The philosophers did not have the same concept of "soul" as we do, and they also did not always use the term *"nous"* in the same way at all times even in their own writings.

15. Epicurus (342-270 B.C.). Appolodorus of Athens "the Chronicler," (d. c. 60 B.C.) Chrysyppos of Soli (280-206 B.C.) was a student of Zeno the Stoic and became head and chief interpreter of the Stoic School. Protagoras the Sophist (490-420 B.C.).

16. We use the word *nous* in all the shades of its meaning since various philosophers had differing concepts of what the hegemonicon consists of.

17. Titus Lucretius Caras (1st Century B.C.) in *On the Nature of Things*, his only surviving poem is a hexametre on the atomic theory of Epicurus. Lucretius held that the soul dies with the body and man becomes extinct at death. He is said to have committed suicide over an unrequited love at the age of about 40.

18. The examples Tertullian used in support of this point ranged from a citation from the *Book of Wisdom* (1:6) where the conscious activity of the intellect and of the will is metaphorically localized in the heart,

107

to the discourse in Matthew's Gospel (5:28) where again the will would seem to be localized in the heart, as adultery is said to be committed there. Strangely, Tertullian seems to have overlooked or ignored the localization of the faculty of memory in the heart clearly implied in Luke's account of Mary's reaction to all that was said and took place (see, for example Lk.2:51).

19. A few references, John Damascene for example, remind us that the soul is created, not a pure spirit, and so it is in some form made of some substance, whether energy or matter (they are the sol and gel of each other).

20. see Puhalo, Lazar, *The Soul, The Body and Death* (Synaxis Press, Dewdney, B.C., 1995) ch.2 and 3. When certain of the holy fathers used the expression "subtle body" to refer to the soul or to angels, they did not have in mind the Gnostic idea of a diaphanous physical body. They wished to make it clear that only God is a "perfect spirit," and that the soul and angels are "created spirits," and so material. They had in mind the imperfect material nature of created spirits. The neo-Gnostic philosopher Fr. Seraphim Rose re-introduced the Gnostic understanding of the phrase into the North American Orthodox Church, to his shame and the grief of many.

21. Wilson, Leonard, *"Erasistratus, Galen, and the Pneuma,"* in Bulletin of the **History of Medicine**, 33, (1959), pp.293-314; Dobson, J.F., *"Erasistratus,"* Proceedings of the Royal Society of Medicine Nr. 20, (London, 1925), pp.825-832; Harris, C.R.S. *The Heart and the Vascular System in Ancient Greek Medicine*, (Oxford, 1973), pp.177-233.

22. One of the problems that arose from the reticence to examine human corpses was the extrapolation of the findings of animal dissection to humans.

23. Galen, *On Anatomical Procedures*, (Charles Singer, London, 1956), Book 9, pp.226-237; Galen, *On Anatomical Procedures, The Later Books,* trans. W.L.H.Duckworth, (Cambridge, 1962), Book 9, pp.1-20; Woollam, D.H.M. *"Concepts of the Brain and its Functions in Classical Antiquity,"* in *The History and Philosophy of Knowledge of the Brain and its Functions*, ed. F.N.L.Poynter, (Oxford, 1958), pp.5-18.

24. *Augustine to Galileo: The History of Science A.D. 400-1650* (Falcon Books, London (1952) p.134-135.

25. Sudhoff, Walther, *"Die Lehre von den Hirnventrikeln in textlicher und graphischer Tradition des Altertums un Mittelalters,"* in **Archiv fur Geschichte der Medizin**, Nr. 7, (1913), pp.149-205.

26. On Bishop Nemesios, see Gilson, Etienne, *Elements of Christian Philosophy,* (Greenwood, Westport, CN., 1979).

27. The heretical teaching that the soul is or has a "subtle body" is purely Gnostic. The concept appeared in a 19th century Russian tract on the soul after death, which was severely condemned by St Theophan the Recluse. To the best of my knowledge, this heresy did not appear again in Orthodox Church writings until it was taken up by the new-Gnostic philosopher Fr Seraphim Rose in his heretical work *The Soul After Death.*

28. Harvey, Ruth, *The Inward Wits—Psychological Theory in the Middle Ages and the Renaissance,* (London, 1975), pp.2-3.

29. Pagel, Walter, *From Paracelsus to Van Helmut: Studies in Renaissance Medicine and Science,* (Vorarium, London, 1986); *Religion and Neo-Platonism in Renaissance Medicine*, in Collected Studies Nr. CS226 (Vorarium, London, 1985).

30. Clarke, Edwain, *An Illustrated History of Brain Function: Imaging the Brain from Antiquity to the Present* (Norman, San Francisco, 1995) 2nd Edn.

31. *On The Resurrection* (Against Origen), 1:5.

32. see for example, St Titus of Bostra, *Homily One, Against the Manicheans,* para.1 (quoted by St John the Damascene: P.G. 96:489B).

33. Gn.2:7; cp. Chapter 1 of this work.

34. P.G. 150, 1361c.

35. *Hymn Eight On Paradise* (complete text in Appendix 1).

36. *Answer 89* (complete text in Appendix 1).

37. The teaching that the soul is a "prisoner of the body," and thus a separate entity which can exit the body, have experiences, receive visions, revelations, wander from place to place, be purged or be "examined and judged" without its body, or indeed, function in any sensual manner without its body is, essentially, pagan Hellenism. Such teachings of the relationship of the body and the soul, called dualism, because they give the soul an actual independent functioning apart from the body, were refuted in the patristic works against Origen and against the Manichean and Gnostic heresies. This doctrine of dualism is also one of the roots of a basic misunderstanding of the dogma of redemption involved in many erroneous teachings. When one penetrates to the essence of such mythologies as purgatory, toll-houses, etc, one finds a basic presupposition that God either cannot or will not forgive sins, but that He must rather obtain some form of satisfaction for them, please Himself with some form of punishment for each transgression. This self-pleasing passion may take the form of physical torment (as in the purgatory myth) or mental and physical torture (as in the toll-house myth). The Latin doctrine of "the saving merits of Christ" is such a teaching also. Here, God does not actually forgive anyone of anything, He only agrees to be satisfied by Christ's suffering, and He is bribed by the excessive merits earned by Christ through His sufferings, and appropriated to a sinner for the sinner's having fulfilled some legal obligation. These teachings of dualism are nearly always bound together with a variation of the "satisfaction theory" of redemption.

38. Some misread Eccl.7:1, "...the day of death is better than the day of one's birth." The Hebrew understanding of this verse is expressed in the Talmudic writings thus: "Why rejoice when a ship leaves harbour and sets forth on a perilous journey: rather rejoice when it safely returns." This also points out the belief in the soul's continuance after death. Taken in connection with related verses and writings, we get a picture of the Old Israel's concept of the nature of the soul and its repose. It is, of course, identical to that of the New Israel, the Orthodox Church, except that the Incarnation and Resurrection of Christ have not only given us a fuller knowledge, but have also changed many things. It is interesting that some people think that the teaching of the Hebrews on this subject should be dramatically different from that of the New Testament Church, as if there were two different Gods, giving two different revelations. The Orthodox Church, after all, is the fulfilled and continued Israel.

39. *On The Resurrection*, chapter 8.

40. Rm.7:24.

41. see St Gregory Palamas, *First Triad*, para.2, answer 2; Methodios of Olympos, *On The Resurrection*, part 1; Fr John Romanides, *The Ancestral Sin*, Athens, 1971.

42. cp. Romanides, *The Nature and Destiny of Man* (Greek Orthodox Theological Review, vol.1, series). Apostle Paul was a Jew, and his concepts and word imagery were Hebraic. The West interpreted Paul with Hellenic, especially Platonic, preconceptions. The meaning of his imagery and even of his words themselves must be related back to Hebrew significations, since Paul was "translating" as it were, Hebrew concepts into Greek, and making do with what words were available.

43. Homily One, *Against the Manicheans*, P.G. 96:489B.

44. *On The Resurrection*, (against Origen), 1:5.

45. e.g., "If a man die, shall he live again? All the days of my appointed time will I wait, till my transformation comes. Thou shalt call, and I will answer Thee: Thou wilt have a desire to the work of Thine hands...If I wait, the grave is my house: I have made my bed in darkness...and where is now my hope...For I know that my Redeemer liveth, and that He shall stand at the latter day upon the earth: and though...worms destroy this body, yet, in my flesh shall I see God: Whom I shall see for myself, and mine eyes shall behold, and not another..." (Jb.14: 14; 17:13; 19:25-26. cp. Jn.5:28-29); "Then shall the dust return to the earth as it was: and the spirit shall return to God Who gave it" (Eccl.12:7); "...the soul shall be bound in the bundle of life with the Lord your God" (1Ki.25:29). "God made man to be immortal, and made him to be an image of His own eternity" (Wis.2:23-24); etc. See also Chapter 3 of this work.

46. This was one of Origen's quandaries once he had adopted the radical dualism of Hellenism and its disdain for the body. He tried to solve it with his theory of "material substratum" (see Chapter 4 of this work). This is also the quandary of the doctrines that souls can be examined and judged at death by demons, aerial toll-houses and the like. Indeed, St Titus of Bostra poses this very question in refuting the radical dualism of the Manicheans (*Homily One*), and Sts Irenae of Lyons and Ambrose of Milan both refute the idea that the soul can be "judged" or physically suffer without the body, in their works against heresies (cited in Appendix A).

47. Sanh.91a, b.

48. *On Belief in The Resurrection*, para.88.

49. Book Five, para.32.

50. Homily One, *Against the Manicheans*, para.1.

51. *Church Synods and Civilisation,* in "Theologica," (July-September, 1992. Athens.) in Greek.

52. *Ascetical Statutes,* c. 18.

53. *Ascetical Statutes,* c. 18.

54. Such amendments to classical medical and scientific theories warn us not to dogmatise patristic writings on these subject. They interpreted the scientific data of their own era in such a way as to accommodate it to Christian doctrine. The scientific data of their era, however, has long since been eclipsed and disproved. The Christian doctrine that they were elucidating has not been. It is as certain now as then.

55. For a life of St Basil the Great, see Puhalo, Lazar, *Great Church Fathers,* (Synaxis Press, Dewdney, B.C., Canada). There are a large number of studies on the life and works of St Basil, from almost every aspect. For the *Hexaemeron,* see the works of St Basil the Great in the Eerdmans' series, *Nicene and Post-Nicene Fathers.*

56. Such an idea is absolutely indispensable to the Gnostic "toll house" myth, reintroduced in our literature by the last neo-Gnostic philosopher Fr. Seraphim Rose.

57. St Gregory of Nyssa, *The Making of Man,* ch. 8-9 and 12 (Nicene and Post Nicene Fathers, Hendrickson, Peabody, Ma.) p. 387 (in P.G., XLIV, cols 144-152, and 155-160.) This is notable, because the Gnostics taught that the body was a prison of the soul, and that the soul, being liberated from the body, experienced new discoveries and rose to its fullest knowledge. The Orthodox Christian Church fathers had precisely the opposite view. Strangely enough, the heretical concept refuted by the holy fathers actually appears in a prayer at the end of the Russian Moleiben for Archangel Michael. This indicates that the prayer was written late in time and warns us to be cautious of forming doctrinal teachings from this particular form of prayer service, many of which were transposed from Latin models.

58. *Teleology:* the interpretation of something in terms of its purpose.

59. Ladner, Gerhardt B., *"The Philosophical Anthropology of Saint St Gregory of Nyssa,"* in the Dumbarton Oaks Papers, 12, (1958), p.69, n.35.

60. see *The Tale of Basil the New* (Synaxis Press, 1998)..

61. Plato, for example, was an adept of Orphic Gnosticism.

62. On Marcion, see Harnack, Adolf, *Marcion, das Evangelium vom fremdem Gott*, (Berlin, 1960) and; Blackman, Edwin C. , *Marcion and his Influence*, (Edwin C. Blackman, London, 1948).

63. On the history of Gnosticism and its relation with other mystery cults Grant, Robert M., *Gnosticism and Early Christianity*, (Columbia University Press, N.Y., 1959); the collection of primary sources, *Gnosticism: A Source Book of Heretical Writers from the Early Christian Period*, Ed. Robert M. Grant, (Columbia University. Press, N.Y., 1961); and Jonas, Hans, *The Gnostic Religion: The Message of the Alien God and the Beginnings of Christianity*,(Peter Smith, Boston, 1963) 2nd rev. ed.

64. For a further study of this Gnosticism, see Puhalo, Lazar, *The Tale of Elder Basil the New: Study of a Gnostic Document* (Synaxis Press, Dewdney, B.C., 1996).

65. See, for example, St Irenae, *Against Heresies,* Bk.4, Ch.6:1; Bk.5, 22;1; 31:2 (Eerdmans, Grand Rapids, 1979) p.309. This same teaching is repeated in almost all the Orthodox Christians refutations of Manichaeism and the other Gnostic heresies. For a study of this theme in the works of St Irenae, see Harnack, Adolf, *Geschichte der altchristlichen Literatur*, (Freiburg im Breisgau, 1913) V.I, pp.263-288.

66. Randall, John Herman Jr. *Hellenistic Ways of Deliverance and the Making of the Christian Synthesis,* (Columbia University Press, New York, 1970), p.161.

67. Harnack, *Medicinisches aus der altesten Kirchengeschichte*, p.6.

68. In this respect, see the extremely important comments of Fr John Romanides in his treatise, *Church Synods and Civilisation*, Theologica, Athens, July-September, 1992.

69. Harnack, Adolph, *Medicinisches aus der altesten Kirchengeschichte*, (Olms, Berlin, 1908) p.2.

70. Harnack, Adolf, *Luke the Physician,* trans. J.R.Wilkinson, (W.D.Morrison, New York, 1908), pp.175-198.

71. Asclepius was the Greek god of medicine. He was likely a practitioner of pre-scientific medicine on the isle of Kos, where Hippocrates was born, and developed a movement toward genuinely

113

scientific medicine.

72. Let us note that psychiatric illnesses are actually physical illness that occur in the brain. Ultimately, we ought not to separate them from the concept of physical illness.

73. Thompson, John D. and Goldin, Grace, *The Hospital: A Social and Architectural History*, (Yale University Press, New Haven, 1975), pp.6 and 327.

74. Acts 6:1-6; Philippians 1:1.

75. See Apostle Paul's commendation of Phoebe at Rm.16:1, and the discussion of women as active servants of the early Church in Harnack, Adolf, *The Mission and Expansion of Christianity*, (Ayer, N. Stratford, NH., 1980).

76. A brief "life" of St Sampson appears in volume 2 of *Lives of Saints for Young People*, Synaxis Press, Dewdney, B.C., Canada. Lives of the other unmercenaries appear in volumes 11, 12 and 13 of the same series.

77. The Emperor Constantine, whose mother Helen devoted her declining years to the establishment of charitable institutions, exercised a decided influence on the Council's deliberations, and Empress Helen was quite interested in the question of the *xenodokhion*. It may be that his consent was necessary for the council's decision to establish a hospital system.

78. Haeser, Heinrich, *Geschichte christlicher Kranken-Pflege und Pflegerschaften*,(Olms, Berlin, 1857) pp.13-15.

79. Haeser, *Geschichte christlicher Kranken-Pflege und Pflegerschaften*, p.17.

80. A life of St Paula may be found in *The Lives of Sts For Young People*, Vol 4; a life of the two Sts Melanie is found in vol. 8 of the same series (Synaxis Press, Dewdney, B.C., Canada). See also the life of St Damian of the Kiev Caves, in *The Kiev Caves Paterikon*, also published in English by Synaxis Press.

81. Galen of Pergamum (A.D.130-200) was the son of the geometer and architect Nikon of Pergamum. As a student of both mathematics and medicine, he studied under Satyrus in Pergamum and, later, the noted physician Pelops in Smyrna. He is one of the most attractive personalities of his time and his writings formed the basis of medicine in Western Europe almost until the Enlightenment. His work was well used among the Byzantine physicians, but they were not bound by them, and progressed beyond him. Among his works were *Diagnosis of Eye Diseases*, *Medical Experience*, *An Anatomy of the Uterus*, and a multitude of important treatises. He may be called the "father of sports medicine," as he served as a physician to gladiators for many years and studied their unique problems. He had a strong prejudice against surgery, which set back his knowledge of internal anatomy somewhat. A critic of the medical school of Alexandria, which he called "scholastic," he nevertheless built on their work. Galen reposed in Pergamum in A.D. 190 or 200.

82. Aulus Cornelius Celsus was a Roman encyclopedist. While he was a prolific writer, only the work *De medicina* survive, because the were preserved by the anti-Gnostic Christians.

83. India was the source of much of the pharmacology of the era. Hindi concepts of pharmacology were certainly known in the school of Jundishapur. Arabic medical research remained bound to alchemy, but made many discoveries and breakthroughs.

84. *Celsus de Medicina*, ed. and trans. W.G.Spenser, 3 vols. (Loeb Classical Library, Harvard University Press, Cambridge, Ma.,1935).

85. Lucius J.M. Columella, who lived in the 1st century, wrote extensively on agriculture. Born in Gades, Spain, he served in the Roman army and later became a farmer, an agriculturist and author of more than 12 books on the subject.

86. Quintilian, the great teacher of rhetoric, was born in Calagori, Spain around A.D.68. He lived and worked in Rome. His *Formation of Oratory* was considered the optimum text on the subject throughout the Middle Ages.

87. Hadas, Moses, *A History of Latin Literature*, (Columbia University Press, New York, 1952), p.239 and, by the same author, *History of Greek Literature* (Columbia University Press, New York, 1950).

88. Origen, *Against Celsus* (Ante-Nicene Fathers, volume 4, Eerdmans, Grand Rapids, 1979). Another excellent English translation of this work is *Origen, Contra Celsus*, ed. Henry Chadwick, (Cambridge, 1953). See also the section on Origen in Chadwick's Early Christian Thought and the Classical Tradition: Studies in Justin, Clement, and

Origen,(Columbia University Press, N.Y., 1966).

89. Origen, *Against Celsus*. Origen deals with this question in several placed. See ch.13 and the following chapters, beginning on p.401 in the Eerdmans edition (Ante-Nicene Fathers, Eerdmans, Grand Rapids, 1974).

90. A few fragments of the agricultural and rhetorical parts have survived. These were edited by Frederick Marx in the first volume of the *Corpus medicorum latinorum*, under the title, *A. Cornelli Celsi quae supersunt*, (Leipzig, 1915).

91. Although most probably not a medical practitioner, Celsus wrote admirably and knew how to select good authorities. Showing special reverence for the Hippocratic writings, he mentioned also more than seventy later medical authors, and his work is our fundamental source for the history of Alexandrian medicine. In the preface to his work, he presented a judicious summary of the history of medicine, and emphasized the advisability of studying natural science as a preparation for medicine.
Celsus' *De medicina,* as the medical section of his work is titled, deals progressively in the first six books with dietetics, diagnosis, prognosis, therapeutics, internal diseases, and pharmacology. Books seven and eight are devoted to surgery and contain anatomical descriptions including a complete account of the skeleton. A masterly compilation, *De medicina* contains many surgical procedures which have become classics such as those describing latter lithotomy, couching the cataract, and removal of the tonsils.

92. *Celsus De Medicina*, tr. W. G. Spenser (Harvard University Press, Cambridge, Ma., 1935).

93. Born at Carthage about 160 A.D., this passionate and violent man was converted to Christianity some thirty years later. Tertullian fell into the heretical sect of the Montanists. Toward the end of his life, however, he rejected Montanism and founded his own heretical sect of the Tertullianists. On Tertullian, see Gilson, Etienne *History of Christian Philosophy in the Middle Ages*, (London, 1955), p.44-46, and pp.574-576; Harnack, Adolf, *The Mission and Expansion of Christianity in the first Three Centuries*, trans. James Moffatt,(London, 1908), II, pp.74-77.

94. Tertullian, strangely enough, believed in the corporality of the soul., See his *Treatise on the Soul*, (Ante-Nicene Fathers, Vol.3, Eerdmans,

116

Grand Rapids, 1975), Ch.5-7.

95. "Atque utinam nullas haereses oportuisset existere, ut probabiles quique emicarent. Nihil omnino cum philosophis super anima quoque experiremur, patriarchis, ut ita dixerim, haereticorum...." In English, Tertullian, *Treatise on the Soul*, Ch. 1-2. in Ante-Nicene Fathers, Vol. 3, pp.181-182 of the Eerdmans' edition.

96. As St Jerome says ,"Quid Tertulliano eruditius, quid acutius? Apologeticus ejus et contra Gentes libri cunctam saeculi continent disciplinam," Epistle 70, 5. (as quoted by Stephen d'Irasay, *"Patristic Medicine,"* in Annals of Medical History, Nr. 9, (1927), p.375.

97. *Treatise on the Soul,* Ch. 15. (The Ante-Nicene Fathers, Vol.3, Eerdman's edition, 1975), pp. 193-194.

98. Nestorius, who died in A.D.451 introduced the heretical notion that Christ had "assumed" His divinity. The Orthodox Christian doctrine holds that Christ assumed our humanity while remaining truly God, and that His humanity and divinity were not mixed or confused. Nestorius' teaching undermined the Gospel of Redemption. After he was deposed as Patriarch of Constantinople, his followers moved to the Eastern regions of the Roman Empire, and into Persia and the area that is now Iraq. They carried with them the Orthodox Christian concepts of medicine and mathematics, and continued the development of medical experimentation and development in the regions the had moved to.

99. Brockelmann, Carl, *History of the Islamic Peoples*, trans. Joel Carmichael (Moshe Perlmann, New York, 1947), pp.124-128.

100. Hitti, Philip K., *The Arabs*, (Gateway, N. Y., 1996), pp.91-92; Meyerhof, Max, *"New Light on Hunain ibn Ishaq* in *Isis*, Vol.8, 1926, pp.685-724.

101. Whipple, A. O., *"The Role of the Nestorians as the connecting link between Greek and Arabic Medicine,"* in Annals of Medical History, 8, n.s. (1936), pp. 313-323.

INDEX

A

B

E

H

N

Q-R

U-Z

LIST OF SCRIPTURE
USED IN THE TEXT

CPSIA information can be obtained
at www.ICGtesting.com
Printed in the USA
LVHW011512120520
655459LV00010B/1406